KW-121-311

UNDER THE KNIFE

SURGICAL STORIES FROM AROUND THE WORLD

Gulzar Mufti

MBBS, MS, MCh, FRCS

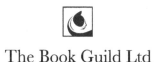

The Book Guild Ltd

First published in Great Britain in 2016 by
The Book Guild Ltd
9 Priory Business Park
Wistow Road, Kibworth
Leicestershire, LE8 0RX
Freephone: 0800 999 2982
www.bookguild.co.uk
Email: info@bookguild.co.uk
Twitter: @bookguild

Copyright © 2016 Gulzar Mufti

The right of Gulzar Mufti to be identified as the author of this
work has been asserted by him in accordance with the
Copyright, Design and Patents Act 1988.

All rights reserved. No part of this publication may be
reproduced, transmitted, or stored in a retrieval system, in any form or by any means,
without permission in writing from the publisher, nor be otherwise circulated in
any form of binding or cover other than that in which it is published and without
a similar condition being imposed on the subsequent purchaser.

Cover Artwork © Ron Hoile MS, FRCS

Typeset in Adobe Garamond Pro

Printed and bound in the UK by TJ International, Padstow, Cornwall

ISBN 978 1910878 828

British Library Cataloguing in Publication Data.
A catalogue record for this book is available from the British Library.

MIX
Paper from
responsible sources
FSC www.fsc.org   FSC® C013056

In loving memory of my mother Tathaji who was my inspiration;
and my father Abbajan who was my leading light

To everyone in my extended family with lots of love and gratitude

Kingston upon Thames Libraries	
KT 2198903 6	
Askews & Holts	04-Jan-2017
617.092 HEA	£8.99
KN	KT00001912

CONTENTS

"Surgeons must be very careful
When they take the knife!
Underneath their fine incisions
Stirs the Culprit—Life!"

EMILY ELIZABETH DICKINSON

FOREWORD

This is a thought-provoking and very readable book and describes some of the many clinical and non-clinical episodes that occurred in the author's much-travelled life, over a varied and successful surgical career. I have known Gulzar for over twenty-five years and had certainly not realised what an amazingly diverse surgical experience he had had (both as patient and surgeon) until I read this book.

For both surgeons and patients a surgical operation is a complex and sometimes frightening experience; albeit for surgeons an oft repeated journey whilst for patients frequently a life changing journey.

The story starts with his place of birth in Srinagar in the Kashmir Valley. He describes his personal experiences with the traditional healers of that time like the barber and the bonesetter and how his early upbringing influenced his career choices. Gulzar then recounts his entry into medical school and how he chose surgery as a career.

The narrative also reports clinical events from colleagues around the world describing their surgical adventures and anecdotes in a wide range of surgical conditions. He also relates some of the trials and tribulations of the frequently inefficient hospital systems and poor management structures he has met across the world trying to draw analogies with modern practice and consider how these thoughts may change practice in the future.

Reading this will allow surgeons to reminisce and reflect on their own practice over the years, which I am sure they will find both highly interesting and highly likely to modify their surgical practice.

There is plenty of description of the importance of learning the technical proficiency of surgery but also clear recognition of the important significance of non-technical skills required, well before their recognition by the many Royal Colleges and their importance in the selection of good surgeons.

The book is written to appeal to both healthcare professionals and the lay public. Some of the additional stories from friends and colleagues may add more for the lay public and certainly add to the readability whilst the dialogue linking them often provides important messages about modern relevance for operating surgeons.

Many of the stories highlight the absolute importance of clear communication in the operating environment and how, without this, things can go badly wrong. It stresses how in the tense operating theatre environment surgeons sometimes do not mean what they say and at other times do not say what they mean. A really good theatre sister is essential!

Not only do these accounts follow the actual surgical events that took place but also describe the great joy and relief that followed some of these procedures.

Whilst there are many anecdotes from the past both from UK and other parts of the world these are regularly related to modern day practice with direct quotes from Royal College of Surgeons and GMC documents such as *Good Medical Practice* showing that the messages from the past are just as relevant today. Gulzar's professional participation in the GMC Fitness to Practise Tribunal work and his knowledge of healthcare regulation through his work with the Care Quality Commission (CQC) also allows him to add useful caveats. It is brought right up to date with recognition of things such as WHO Surgical checklists (based on airline pilot checks) and the UK avoidance of '*Never Events*' such as retained surgical instruments and wrong side surgery, steps which the good surgeons of the past took without realising they were doing many of them.

There is much we can all learn from this novel as it charts both a personal journey and to an extent the development of modern surgical and urological practice.

Whilst this book would make a good holiday read, it could alternatively be dipped into at the end of a busy day just to pick out individual chapters all of which have clear titles such as; *The Apprentice, Communication, When things go wrong* and *Gratitude and Trust.*

Mark J Speakman
President
British Association of Urological Surgeons
April 2016

INTRODUCTION

To deliberately thrust a knife or any sharp object into another human being is profound. Blood will flow. Done by an assailant, the intention of course is to harm and cause pain. It will kill or maim. But in the hands of a skilled surgeon, a finely honed blade can save life, dramatically improve the quality of existence, relieve pain, get rid of threatening intrusions, and correct disabling disfigurements. Whilst an assailant speedily quits the scene of crime, the surgeon stays around to supervise recovery and care – in some cases for a long time thereafter. Unlike the attacker, a surgeon never uses the scalpel without seeking permission and there is a shared intention to heal, to cure ailments or at least improve the quality of life.

I have been using knives and other surgical instruments on people for more than forty years with the best possible motives, of course. The overwhelming majority of my patients lived to tell the tale. Tragically, there are some who didn't, despite the best efforts of the surgical team. As I ruminate about my years I feel that a surgical career is like a safari that takes you through a beautiful and enjoyable landscape and throws at you delights, surprises and challenges of all kinds. Along the way you run into a variety of creatures – big as well as small, mighty as well as meek, crafty as well as candid, of all shapes and forms – colleagues, peers, juniors and bosses. More importantly, you meet tens of thousands of patients and their loved ones. The healthcare managers of twenty-first century describe these encounters as 'clinical episodes'.

Every such episode – in fact every event that occurs in the healthcare environment, is a story. We clinicians are unique in the sense that in our day-to-day working lives stories are narrated all the time, in clinics, operating theatres, hospital corridors, GP surgeries, and in fact at any place where clinical activity takes place.

Many clinical stories from the world of surgery are reported and talked about in scientific journals in different forms such as: clinical research papers, case reports, and letters to the editor. Some are highlighted in the print, electronic and social media in the form of news items, articles, opinion pieces, magazine columns, blogs and so forth. Some are a favourite theme for the television and radio industry. However, there is also a large pool of interesting anecdotes – clinical and non-clinical, embedded in the memory banks of the professionals involved. These are narrated to close audiences in clinicians' gatherings and social get-togethers, when colleagues share these during informal chats. There are many more that are never shared and remain untold.

In my working lifetime I was personally involved with numerous clinical and non-clinical events, some of which were interesting enough to occupy a permanent space in my memory closet. Over the years I also heard many fascinating stories from my senior and junior colleagues. I made a note of some of them. For this book I also contacted surgeons in many parts of the world with the request to dig deep into their memory banks and recall interesting episodes of their clinical life. I emphasised to them that the content needed to be factual and not too scientific or specialised. It was encouraging to receive a variety of anecdotes from a range of individuals from many countries, covering different time periods. So I was able to accumulate a collection over a period of time.

From the large pool of collected material, I selected the stories that appear in this book. After taking into account various confidentiality issues, each story was tailored to a uniform editorial style but I made sure that the core theme of the incident or event was not distorted. In order to respect the confidentiality of individuals involved, where necessary, patients' as well as clinicians' initials were changed and locations altered.

Some of the stories and events described in the book are light-hearted and hilarious, some are unexpected, heroic, or even miraculous, some are awkward or embarrassing, and some are painful, tragic or even disastrous, but all are factual: so what you read is essentially all true. Whilst the majority of episodes conclude in a satisfactory or a cheerful outcome with smiles all round, a few have unfavourable, sad or even catastrophic endings. But each anecdote is a source of experience for all those involved and for all others who hear about them.

This book, however, is not a collection of stories but much like illustrations in a textbook, selected anecdotes have been used to lace together and amplify the narrative. Each story makes a small point and when you join the points you create the big picture. The purpose is take the reader on a walkabout through the day-to-day happenings and the highs and lows of the world of surgery, and to provide an insight into the persona of surgeons – their feelings and emotions, their strengths and weaknesses, their joys and sorrows, their dreads and delights and more. Moreover, the book is about patients who put their life into the hands of a surgeon. It also explores various facets of patient-surgeon relationship including public perceptions about surgeons.

The public view about surgery in general and surgeons in particular is shrouded in contradiction. Whilst phrases like action and excitement, valour and heroism, commitment and dedication, skill and knowledge, expertise and experience are acknowledged; words like egoism, grandeur, power and authority are also linked with the occupation. The accounts of surgical accidents reported prominently in the media in recent times not only raised public awareness about safety and quality in surgical practice, but also dented the surgical image to some extent. The debate that followed helped to strengthen the processes of professional and healthcare regulation in the West. Despite the alarms, in actual fact the vast majority of surgeons are highly skilled, competent, hardworking and caring professionals. For them the sole purpose of being a surgeon is the welfare of their patients. Some of them work in trying conditions and some battle their way through inefficient hospital systems and poor management structures. This book is meant as a tribute to the surgical fraternity worldwide who are constantly subjected to the vicissitudes of surgical life.

Gulzar Mufti
Maidstone, Kent, England
May 2016
gulzar.mufti@gmail.com

1

THE BEGINNING

Technological and scientific advances of recent years have revolutionised the surgical craft with the result that procedures and treatments that were considered too complex or impracticable in the past became a daily routine. For a surgeon like me with many miles on the clock it has been a fascinating experience to watch, or in some cases be involved at close range with the evolution and development of such advancements, but the pleasure is all the more when I sit back to reminisce and reflect, before the shadows of twilight set in and blur the exit points of my memory cabinet.

At the dawn of my medical career I could certainly not have imagined that I would be able to fish out a stone from a patient's kidney without cutting into the body, or I would be removing human urinary bladders affected by diseases like cancer and would be replacing them with new bladders made from patients' own bowels, and that the reconstructed organ would function nearly as well as the natural one. Nor could I conceive then that surgeons would be able to remove large diseased body organs, growths or unwanted objects through small holes; that after death a single human would be able to donate purposeful life to many others; and that robotic hands would in due course take over surgical craftsmanship from humans.

Such exploits are a far cry from my early days, growing up in the foothills of Himalayas in the panoramic Kashmir Valley, described by British civil servant Sir Walter Lawrence as *an emerald set in pearls*. I was born and brought up in Srinagar, also known as the Venice of Asia, which is the capital of Kashmir Valley, at the time when the subcontinent was going through the after effects of the agony and bloodshed of Partition.

I was lucky to be born in a family where education was a priority and was given a brisk start by my mother who worked as a teacher in a public school. She was one of the first literate ladies of the state, and was educated in an era when sending girls to school was considered unthinkable. My father was a revenue magistrate who also came from the educated element of Kashmiri society.

British Christian missionaries had brought to this land English education and western system of medicine during the late nineteenth century, the benefits of which were reaped by generations – including me. Two famous surgeon brothers Arthur and Ernest Neve established the first hospital – the Kashmir Mission Hospital, and Cecil Tyndale-Biscoe and Muriel Mallinson founded high schools of international repute for boys and girls respectively.

I started my schooling in the 1950s. By then the seeds of education sown by the British missionaries at the beginning of the twentieth century had already borne fruit. The streets of Srinagar used to be crowded with boys and girls from all social strata during school opening and closing times. Despite the outwardly calm, there was tension in the air; a state of cold war existed between two newly independent countries: India and Pakistan – for both Kashmir was the unfinished business of Partition.

Prior to the introduction of the western school of medicine in the Valley by the first Scottish missionary doctor from Aberdeen, Dr William Elmslie, the responsibilities of healthcare were shared amongst traditional care providers of that era: the *hakím* (physician), the *dirke-gor* (leech applier), the *naevid* (barber), the *wáttan-gor* (bone setter) and the *wáren* (midwife). All except the last of these were exclusively male occupations. The *wáren* was the wise old lady of the locality who diagnosed a pregnancy and looked after antenatal, natal and postnatal care. She conducted the delivery in patients' homes.

As a lad it was fascinating to watch my father's cousin and one of my favourite uncles – a professional *hakím*, conducting his private clinic at his home. By early morning his dark and dingy consultation room would become jam-packed with patients and their carers, except for a triangular area in the top corner that was reserved for him. Everyone sat on the floor and after the boss' arrival each patient would slowly wriggle up the queue with an outstretched arm. After a question or two my uncle would feel a patient's radial pulse, write a prescription and offer advice about what not to drink and eat. The consultation would conclude within a minute or two.

Hakíms were the modern day non-interventionist physicians who practised the Greek-Arabian system of Medicine and laid a lot of emphasis on dietetic restrictions as part of the treatment regimen. For instance, no solid foods were allowed for acute illnesses, particularly those associated with fever. They believed the cause of sickness to be unhealthy blood and prescribed bloodletting as a treatment for serious cases and would therefore recruit the services of a *dirke-gor* (leech-therapist) who used leeches to suck blood from the individual. The *hakím* would, however, mark the vein to be used for that purpose.

The section of the Hippocratic Oath (classical version) mandating, '*I will not use the knife, not even on sufferers from stone, but will withdraw in favour of such men as are engaged in this work*' was followed scrupulously by a Kashmiri *hakím*. He did not dip into surgical waters but left that to a *naevid* who combined surgery with his main job of shaving and cutting hair; much like the European surgeons of the Middle Ages who were also barbers and combined their haircutting expertise with surgery, like amputations.

3

A Kashmiri barber's tool-kit comprised a sharp razor with a wooden handle that would normally be used for shaving the scalp or face and for making the edges of beard or moustache, a pair of scissors, pliers, hooks and wires of various types. The procedures included dental extractions; fixation of loose teeth, removal of earwax and drainage of abscesses, but the commonest operation performed by a barber was circumcision on Muslim boys for religious reasons, which used to be a ceremonial occasion for the whole family.

During my boyhood days healthcare was in a transition stage; modern techniques had come in and a 400-bed state funded, modern hospital had been commissioned, but old-fashioned methods of treatment were still being practised widely, particularly in villages. Due to the dearth of qualified doctors, even in towns and cities barbers and other non-qualified personnel enjoyed profitable medical and surgical practices. Since the vast majority of populace was Muslim there was a lucrative market for circumcisions and several practitioners had acquired fame for their expertise in this field. I have a hazy memory of my encounter at close quarters with one of them during the early 1950s.

My younger brother and I were the centre of attention as friends and relatives started gathering at our family home. After a warm bath we were dressed up in newly stitched outfits and led into the largest room of our family home, which was full of relatives. Green tea and a variety of baked goods were being served and everyone in the room was cheering and singing. I can recall a shower of kisses landing on my cheeks as I was led into the nearby room wearing a long shirt. Completely unaware of what was going on, I was coaxed down onto a mattress on the floor. Held and kept amused by a few people, with one stroke of a razor the circumciser detached the foreskin and followed it with firm application of cloth held by thread. There was a loud cheer all round.

I still remember clearly the man's face – his neatly trimmed beard and large black eyes peering through his round glasses. I cannot recollect feeling any pain or crying during the procedure but can recall my brother and I waddling carefully around the house afterwards. The pain was intense when the dry and hardened dressing was taken off a week or so later.

A Kashmiri *wáttan-gor* (bonesetter) largely dealt with orthopaedic trauma; his field of expertise ranged from a minor sprain to a broken spine. As a boy I had the opportunity of witnessing the *modus operandi* of a well-known bonesetter of that era.

On a warm drizzly morning after a sluggish walk of about half a mile through dusty narrow lanes of downtown Srinagar, my dad and I ambled into a large dark room on the ground floor of a brick built house. This was the consulting chamber of the expert on bone trauma. An old man with a long snowy white beard, emotionless face and a massive white turban was seated on a shabbily carpeted floor at the top end of the room, with a large oblong pillow supporting his back. The master was busy applying rolled cloth to a young man's leg that was being supported by two well-built men who were the patient's family members.

The expert greeted my dad courteously and asked us to be seated on the floor. After finishing the job in hand he directed us to move closer to him. After exposing his swollen right hand and forearm that was being supported by his own left hand, my dad narrated the story to the old man.

"Two days ago I was travelling by horseback when suddenly my horse went crazy and threw me off his back – the horse probably hit a sharp stone and both he and I fell." My dad's job involved travelling from one town or village to another – at that time some of the places were poorly connected by vehicular transport.

Without saying much the bonesetter started cutting a few pieces of cloth and cardboard, following which he held my dad's hand and began prodding it. Then he asked one of the attendants of his previous patient to hold my dad's forearm firmly near the elbow. He gripped the swollen and painful hand and fingers firmly in his right hand and pulled it hard, with the assistant offering counter-traction at the elbow. I could see that there was still a lot of strength in the old man as he matched the counter-pull by a much younger and muscular individual. My dad groaned in agony, turned pale and sweaty with pain, and almost passed out. I remember hearing a grating sound coming from the injured part.

The trauma specialist applied the first principle of fracture management i.e.: traction and followed it by the second i.e.: immobilisation, for which he fixed a strip of cardboard on my dad's hand and part of his forearm. Over that he applied a long strip of rolled cloth, and finally he placed the traumatised arm in a large rectangular white cotton sling, that was held by a knot around the neck.

During the whole episode the elderly man didn't speak – nor did he flicker, but for the little fellow accompanying the patient the episode was a distressing as well as a tearful experience.

After paying the dues my dad and I started our lumbered return walk home, with my hand holding his normal hand. I wanted to cry but didn't and broke the silence by asking, "Does it hurt?"

"Yes, a little bit, but you have got to be brave." He replied with a broad smile. And that made me feel better.

As a boy I had an indirect encounter with a Kashmiri *wáren* (midwife) too. A middle-aged lady covered in a white *burqa* (a loose pleated white robe of Afghani origin) arrived in the morning at my parental home in downtown Srinagar. She was taken by my grandma into the smallest room in the house where my mum was lying on a bed. After staying for about half an hour the lady departed; it was probably too early for her expertise to be put to test. As the night fell my mother's screams became louder. A messenger was despatched to fetch the midwife who arrived promptly – and this time she decided to stay. As I woke up next morning I could hear my mum's periodic shrieks, which eventually stopped just before midday. I can distinctly recall the lady leaving at that time as my grandma handed over to her cash and goods in kind.

After her departure a state of gloom engulfed our happy home for many days, with all family elders crying and sobbing at periodic intervals. My mother had lost the baby during prolonged childbirth. A life had ended before it had begun. Silence prevailed in our home for many weeks thereafter.

The foregoing experiences involving pseudo-surgeons – traditional healers who dabbled in various tributaries of surgery – were traumatic but while still at school I was lucky to meet real surgeons too. The first opportunity was when on our way home from my school my dad decided to drop by the local hospital in Srinagar to visit a young relative who had undergone a surgical operation.

The boy in his early teens was lying on a bed in a single room that had been allocated to him because his dad was a high-ranking Government official. The room was crowded and noisy with a large number of relatives and friends.

"His testis was in the wrong place and was repositioned by an operation." I overheard an elderly man informing my dad.

"Who performed the operation?" asked my dad.

"Dr G ... he has recently returned from England, he is FRCS. They say he is very bright."

The dialogue was interrupted suddenly by the imposing entry of a tall, broad-shouldered and overweight gentleman in his early forties with a distinctively large belly. He was Dr G who had been the subject of conversation between the stranger and my dad. With his impressive entry there was a sudden lull and all present stood up to attention.

Dr G went to the patient's bedside, lifted the red bed blanket, and after examining the young lad turned round, and with a broad smile announced in a thick husky voice, "Good, everything is fine. We will discharge him from the hospital tomorrow." With that statement he made an equally rapid exit, and after that the noise in the room returned – on a much louder scale.

The whole episode was quick – the gentleman broke into a scene and went out like lightning. "He must be a very important person!" I thought to myself.

The second episode with a real surgeon was a couple of years later, when my dad was admitted to the only private hospital in Srinagar with a surgical diagnosis. The whole family – my mother, grandmother, uncles and aunts – were waiting in the hospital corridor for a meeting with the surgeon Dr P. Being the eldest child in the family I was there too.

Dr P was a UK-trained surgeon, a close look-alike of the famous Hollywood actor Cary Grant – handsome young man with an aura and dressed immaculately in a neatly tailored double-breasted blue suit. He arrived briskly at the appointed time and everyone stood in quiet attention. He made his way into the room through the waiting crowd. From a distance I watched him speak to my dad by his bedside. After looking at the X-ray films he came out of the room into the corridor and explained the details of my dad's illness to the waiting crowd. In an assured but kind and compassionate manner he announced the verdict, "He needs a major operation to remove the kidney stone and I will perform that later in the week."

"Could he lose the kidney, sir?" asked one of my older uncles.

"Yes sir, he could," Dr P replied confidently.

"Could the operation pose a danger to his life, sir?" enquired my grandmother.

"Yes madam, it could. That danger is always there. You see we are talking of a very big operation," came his prompt reply.

There was a hush all round and after a couple of supplementary questions Dr P made a brisk exit. And then the noisy debate began. Everyone went into the room where my dad was admitted. All were satisfied with the way Dr P had explained everything and praised his bedside manner and courtesy. They talked about the operation and the use of the anaesthetic liquid with a mask. "Would he wake up after that?" My uncle asked. "…Besides, Dr P clearly said that there was a real risk of death," stated my grandma.

At the end it was agreed unanimously that an operation was out of the question. A discharge was requested; opinions were sought from the best physician in town who prescribed injections and pills, and from a leading *hakim* who was well known for prescribing the stone dissolving mixture – the recipe for which had apparently been passed on to him from his father. Thanks to the potpourri of prayers, prescriptions and pills, remarkably my father's symptoms improved but the problem persisted for many decades thereafter – in actual fact, as long as he lived.

By the time I became eligible for admission to medical school I was firm in my resolve to choose Medicine as a career. I cannot pinpoint the reasons for that but it was a delight for me to be invited for the interviews to compete for a place. The occasion brought me face-to-face with the famous Dr R – the father of modern surgery in Kashmir. He was the first Kashmiri surgeon to acquire the qualification of FRCS, first to use the wonder drug penicillin on Kashmiri patients, and the first to perform prostatectomy (removal of prostate) in Kashmir.

Dr R had recently retired from the post of chief surgeon and administrator at the local hospital and was known to be a safe and skilled surgeon. He was also famous for his discipline. It was said that he would never speak loudly to anyone – his look was apparently enough. His operating theatre list would always start on the dot – a late arriving staff member would prefer to send in a leave application and return home rather than be seen arriving late. I had also heard that he was ambidextrous, and that he prayed before starting each case in theatre.

I was naturally nervous but determined to do well. Dressed in a pink poplin shirt with well-oiled and tidily combed scalp hair, I entered the room and saw Dr R seated in a chair towards the left of the room – stern and stocky and neatly bearded, with a rather rigid face and a long and pointed chin with scarce hair growth. The thinly built, squinted but smiling panel chairman made me comfortable and after a couple of straightforward questions passed me on to Dr R.

As he fixed his gaze on me over his round and wiry spectacles I felt like a mouse in trap; and a chill ran through my spine. His chin started moving and out came the question in a soft but loud voice.

"Why do you want to be a doctor?"

"Sir, I want to serve the poor." These were the exact words that I had been coached to reply.

"And not the rich?" he enquired.

I was disarmed completely. That was certainly not in my script. Being a few years younger and therefore much smaller in size than my fellow competitors I felt like poor Mowgli from the film *Jungle Book* – the man cub in front of the mighty Shere Khan (without the glittering nails!). I waffled round in circles whilst Dr R continued with his unblinking, ice-cold expression but somehow I managed to keep out of reach of his tiger-like claws.

"No more questions from me," he turned towards the Chairman, who in turn lifted my spirits by uttering a neat and decisive thank you. The rest of the interview continued without much difficulty.

As I left the room I felt good – released from a grip, but more importantly I had just met the great man about whom I had heard so much. Despite my own perception of being unable to withstand the torment of Dr R's penetrating gaze the committee judged me suitable for admission to the medical school.

So there I was – one amongst the sixty-six entrants from diverse backgrounds bundled together by fate, and destined to spend more than five years of our youth together.

The first two years were spent in studying anatomy on dead humans in the dissection hall, and physiology in classrooms and laboratories learning how a human being functions. However, as we moved from the cadaveric world into clinical lane life became livelier and fast-paced. It brought us in contact with people of all kinds – patients, public and all those who keep the wheels of healthcare on the move. That included doctors from all disciplines – anatomists, laboratory experts, researchers, academics, physicians and surgeons from different specialties.

One day followed another and as months rolled into years we developed and grew together, both physically and mentally, and matured into youthful adults. The vast majority of us metamorphosed into doctors.

Medical school years are truly memorable. They lay the foundations of many lifelong friendships. As we left our mother hen – the medical school – like a cluster of seeds, the winds of destiny scattered us in different directions. And that was the beginning of a long and adventurous journey for each one of us.

2

TYING THE KNOT

As the excitement of qualifying as a doctor starts waning away, it is time for the young medical graduate to reflect and make an important decision – choose a specialty for a future career. For those who pick surgery as the favourite option, the question lurking in the background is: what attributes should a wannabe possess to become a surgeon?

An old English aphorism assumes that a good surgeon has an eagle's eyes, a lady's hands and a lion's heart. But does every surgeon have all these virtues, and does the absence of any of these qualities rule you out from taking surgery as a career? A good pair of eyes is fine but 3D digital technology and fibre optics have transformed the visual landscape of surgery. Besides, it is not uncommon to come across surgeons with massive hands who perform surgical procedures like artwork. I have also witnessed roaring surgical personalities crack under pressure when the going got tough. Having said that the adage is probably relevant conceptually – good surgeons are sharp observers, have a soft touch when handling tissues and possess good leadership qualities.

The Royal College of Surgeons (RCS) of England entices young medical students and graduates to take up surgery as a career stating that *anyone can become a surgeon if they are willing*

12

to work hard towards their career. However, it cautions that *the training can be lengthy and requires commitment*. The Royal College of Surgeons of Edinburgh advises that: *To succeed, you will need to be determined and enthusiastic and have a passion for the specialism that you wish to pursue. You will need to be self-motivated and emotionally stable, possess good decision-making skills and be cool and calm under pressure.*

The guidance from the American College of Surgeons is somewhat similar. It counsels the young hopeful to *appreciate working as a member of a team; enjoy watching your patients improve daily after major injuries or surgical procedures; embrace responsibility and the opportunity to make a positive impact; excel at problem solving and have the ability to "think on your feet"; feel intrigued by the challenge of managing multiple physiological and psychological problems in your critically ill surgical patients; share the excitement of a surgical team anticipating a "great case"; enjoy the challenges of acquiring new technical skills and understanding new technologies.*

I have asked a number of friends and colleagues – trainees as well as established surgeons, the reasons for selecting surgery as an occupation. For the majority it was the ambition of their life, but a small number admitted that they came into it by chance. I also used to ask this question to prospective applicants for surgical training jobs during the course of interviews and have heard interesting replies such as: "I love the thrill of surgery." "I love action." "My thinking has always been surgical." "Surgeons don't mess about, they get on with the job in hand." "I think I am a good leader and that is what a surgeon should be." "I am good with my hands;" and so on. However, the most bizarre answer I heard was during my early years as a consultant in the UK National Health Service (NHS).

I was one of the four members of an interview panel appointing for three vacant positions of senior house officers (junior surgical trainees/residents). Seven candidates had been invited for the interview. The next candidate to come into the room was the sixth

13

person on the list – we had already interviewed five. The candidate had a good CV; had qualified with honours and had published a couple of papers in medical journals. He was one of the favourites to be appointed to one of the posts. As he came in, the Chairman directed him towards the waiting chair and introduced him to panel members, and then the interview began.

The tall and stiff looking man appeared nervous, which was understandable, but apart from being brief there was nothing unusual about the answers that he gave to the questions by first three panel members – the questions were straightforward and matter of fact and so were the answers. And then came my turn and I asked him my favourite question, "Why do you want to be a surgeon?"

He fixed his gaze at me whilst he was thinking of an answer, and after a prolonged and embarrassing silence, with an expressionless face and without a blink in his eyes he said, "Because," and following another protracted pause added, "I love the sight of blood." When I pressed him to tell me why that was so, he responded with a stiff stare and a stony silence. That was frightening enough for everyone on the panel to rule him out for the job.

After he left the panel members looked at one another. No one said anything until the Chairman broke the silence, "Did you notice that he was wearing a jet black shirt – a spooky colour to wear for an interview, I guess?"

The RCS website incorporates comments by surgeons that explain the reasons for choosing a surgical career. These include: surgery being a challenging and rewarding career in which practical skill and creativity can be nurtured, having a personality that thrives on obtaining fairly instant results, and having 'an inkling' and the 'urge to tinker and fix.'

At the time of my own decision-making my thoughts were clear. I did not wish to be a GP and I knew I could not handle screaming women in labour. As a medical student I had managed to undertake a single normal delivery, observed a single forceps delivery and assisted in a single Caesarean Section. I could not take any more of that.

Nor could I bear seeing a child in pain and distress, and I wasn't sure how doctors could make decisions by listening to a shrieking child's chest through a stethoscope. I might as well be a vet! As far as I was concerned I had two choices: either medicine or surgery. Was I going to be the thoughtful physician in a white coat with a long hanging stethoscope, and write prescription after prescription after careful analysis of symptoms and signs, or was I going to make a living by cutting into fellow human beings?

Even though deep down I did not fancy the first option I had an open mind and had a few queries with no clear answers. During my surgical posting as a medical student, I had a few opportunities of going into an operating theatre. However, we had strict instructions to maintain a fair distance from the field of action – the operating table. All we were able to see was a group of people huddled around an unconscious human, moving their hands and arms in different directions.

My parents were not particularly warm to the idea of me becoming a surgeon. My dad used to rub shoulders with doctors and was well versed with the acronym MRCP (Member of Royal College of Physicians) – these letters made his face glow with excitement and anticipation. He had wished all along that I acquired these letters after my name. When I floated the idea that I might train to become a surgeon, he wasn't entirely pleased and I remember him advising me: "You want to be a surgeon – rip and repair – that is your choice but you need to think carefully…"

Despite my inclination for surgery some questions still bothered me. Apart from the ability to read and assimilate books on surgery, what else did I need to become a surgeon? Did I possess the dexterity to cut, to stitch, separate tissues and so on? Did I have the personality to lead with self-belief and courage, and most importantly was I brave enough to make cuts on live human beings to alleviate suffering and pain? And was there anything else that I needed in addition to these qualities? One thing was sure though: I did not have the bulky physique, and rich, thick and thunderous voice of Sir Lancelot Spratt, as depicted in the *Doctor* series of English films of 1960s. With no career guidance available in those days, the choice had to be mine. But how the final decision was made is a story in itself.

The last three months of my six months' compulsory internship – before I could be registered as a doctor, were in a general surgery unit, to work for a careful, but carefree, larger than life general surgeon, Professor K, who knew how to enjoy life to the full. On my first day in the unit I was ordered to go to theatre and scrub (wash both hands and forearms) as the second assistant with the boss. As I finished scrubbing to put on the theatre gown, the head theatre assistant (equivalent of a theatre manager) – who was timing me quietly at a distance without my knowledge – ordered me to scrub again, because I had not washed for full ten minutes. The tension that was already building inside me and which I was trying to hide intensified further. However, my registrar who was scrubbing under a tap next to mine, and who was going to be the first assistant, noticed my anxious body language and calmed me down. "Relax, you are going to be fine," he said reassuringly.

The rather bulky Prof K was going to operate on a rather bulky lady patient for open cholecystectomy (removal of gall bladder). I was directed to stay on the left side of the surgeon. As he made one long vertical cut in the upper part of the patient's abdomen he and the registrar picked up all small bleeding vessels meticulously one by one by applying a row of clips, and started ligating each one of these with catgut (absorbable thread made from a sheep's bowel). The registrar cut the ends of the first two ligatures, and then handed over the scissors to me. Using both hands and my total concentration I tried to keep pace with the boss and his first assistant and cut the ligatures in exactly the same manner as the registrar had done. The boss cautioned me gently, twice, by saying, "Not too short boy, not too short!"

As soon as Prof K's hands went inside the patient's abdomen, he handed over to me a broad steel retractor. After placing it carefully under the patient's right chest wall he asked me to pull to give him a good exposure of the abdominal cavity. I could not see what was going on in there but the three of them – scrub nurse included – managed to pluck the gall bladder out whilst I received a few hard nudges from Prof K's left elbow. Each time he reminded me not to release my tight grasp on the retractor.

The atmosphere relaxed as soon as the gall bladder was delivered and Prof K began suturing the abdominal wall layer by layer. As he started putting in the first stitch through the last layer of abdominal wall (skin), the registrar had to leave to see a patient on the ward. Prof K appeared bored and all of a sudden he too decided to leave the table. As he walked off, without even looking at me, in a husky voice he commanded, "Suture the skin, doctor."

My heart started galloping as I looked helplessly at the male scrub nurse who smiled at me and said, "Come on, we will be fine – do it exactly the same way as he did for the first stitch."

Holding a toothed dissecting forceps and a straight sharp cutting needle attached to a long black silk thread, gradually but confidently I worked my way through the long incision and applied a row of vertical mattress sutures. As I was putting in the last stitch I realised that Prof K and the head theatre assistant – who had ordered me to scrub again, were talking to each other near the theatre door and were also watching the proceedings. I realised that my needlework was being scrutinised; clearly Prof K had been making sure that I did not make a mess.

I felt a sigh of enjoyable relief that the procedure was over and that I had come through it successfully. My exit from the operating theatre was somewhat blocked by Prof K and the head theatre assistant standing close to the door and therefore I decided to stand uneasily nearby, when the head theatre assistant started a conversation with me.

"Did you enjoy the operation?"

My honest reply was, "Yes, I did."

"You should become a surgeon," he said in an authoritative manner.

"Do you really think so?" I asked hesitatingly.

"Yes, I do," he replied.

Prof K joined the conversation at this point and said, "I agree..." and after giving me a long piece of advice about the challenges of being a surgeon he concluded by saying, "Remember, the only thing that the patient sees are the stitches on the skin."

Both these men had made my day. I felt chuffed. I had put in a neat row of skin sutures in a confident manner and had received endorsement not only from Prof K but from the head theatre assistant, who was a daunting personality in his own right and who was well known within the organisation – adored by some and despised by some, but respected by all. After all he had worked in that theatre for thirty years with hundreds of juniors and seniors, including the famous Dr R who had interviewed me for admission to the medical school.

A decision about my future had been made. With the help of these two individuals I had tied the knot for life – I was going to be a surgeon; I was going to learn to use a knife on fellow humans to heal and to cure. Perhaps I was lucky to meet two great men with vast surgical experience who facilitated my entry into the surgical arena, which was undoubtedly the best decision of my life.

I made that choice a few decades ago. Since then the world has moved on. New methodologies like aptitude assessment, cognitive testing, simulation-based surgical skills laboratories and other processes have been introduced to assess the suitability of an applicant for surgical training. Evidence suggests that technical proficiency skill testing helps to choose an applicant with the aptitude for surgery. As surgery becomes more and more complex and sophisticated, and as new techniques and technology emerge, it is now accepted that surgical expertise is attained through continuous training, practice and education. In-born talent does play a role but is probably insufficient on its own to produce a surgical expert. In the modern era the old maxim – surgeons are born not made – does not hold water any more.

3

THE APPRENTICE

A zeal of zebras on a fast gallop, a flock of birds on a frisky flight or a parade of elephants on a lethargic walkabout – these are the typical sights encountered on a jungle safari. A trip along a long and generally crowded hospital corridor is not too different. You could run into a bunch of nurses marching merrily in a rhythmic formation, a committee of managers – with jumbled notebooks and Filofaxes held close to their chest walls – sprinting from one meeting to another, a group of well-built and uniformed security personnel on a leisurely walkabout, and various other staff groups with distinguishing outfits and identities. Amongst them you might also find clusters of doctors pacing briskly in both directions – on their rounds – on their way to see patients on another ward or floor or wing of the hospital.

Rounds (known as ward rounds in some places) undertaken by surgeons are short and brisk, thus the joke amongst physicians that a surgeon's round is a walk-about; some call it a leap-about. On the other hand rounds by physicians are slow paced, time-consuming and detailed – some surgeons would say long-winded and repetitive. Going round a twenty-bed ward can take them hours. I asked one of my physician friends why they took so long to finish a ward round. His response was quite measured and physician like: "Our ward round is like your operating theatre – we sneak inside a human body – through a window or even a chink in a window, that is why we take our time; you guys bang open the door!"

In the past a team of doctors would traditionally start their rounds from the hospital ward or floor belonging to that unit or department. The ward sister or charge nurse would greet the head of the team, and after exchanging pleasantries the ward doors would be shut, and the medical and nursing staff would move from one bed to another visiting one patient after another. In many countries the routine is still the same, but due to an overall decrease in bed numbers in the UK the scenario has changed, nowadays one finds patients scattered all over the hospital on different wards and locations.

As a general rule Surgery has a vertical organisational structure and the person at the apex of the pyramid has the final say in decision-making. Known by one of the many titles like Chief, Prof, Sir, Don – or as Mr, Miss, Madam, Mrs or Doctor – usually followed by the surname or simply the first letter of the surname, the individual is easily distinguishable from the rest by the air of authority. The head-boy or head-girl – known as the senior registrar or chief resident, is seen walking humbly alongside, and along with the ward sister does most of the talking with the boss. The rest of the entourage generally open their mouths only when required.

There are layers of authority between the boss at the top and the youngster at the bottom of the ladder who has just made entry into the surgical world. Depending on the country of practice there could be a few associate/assistant professors, lecturers, registrars, fellows, residents, senior or junior house officers in the pack. They all are at different stages of their training or seniority. The bigger the firm, the bigger the boss and it is not unusual to find a large group of people working for a professor in a big teaching hospital. For the junior, a smaller firm is generally better because there are fewer bosses and more practical handiwork to do. But it is also necessary for the apprentice to work in larger centres with the experts in individual crafts. That serves the purpose of an icing on a cake and also provides an opportunity to get to know the bigwigs in the trade.

It is not uncommon to hear the phrase 'a well-run surgical firm' which means a surgical unit with a good disciplinary code of practice down the line – similar to the military. In the past most surgeons were called to serve in the military and were involved with action in the battlefield, where the working practice required a decisive chief officer and an effective chain of command. The style and some of the hierarchical patterns of authority so observable in surgical practice and training owe something to surgery's connection with the military. In both vocations directives are relayed down the chain and in most cases the expected outcome is compliance.

Many years ago I was scheduled to meet a company boss – a non-medico, in London. He was late for the appointment and when he eventually arrived for the meeting, amidst a shower of apologies he said, "Actually the reason for being late is that I had to visit my son who has been admitted to the hospital with abdominal pain."

"Is he okay?" I asked as a matter of courtesy.

"Yes, he is. I had to wait for the surgeon under whom he is admitted to tell me what is wrong with him; I was there when the commander came round with his crew. He put his hand on my son's tummy and announced: 'acute appendicitis; to theatre; first on the list' and walked off."

I wasn't surprised to hear the military phraseology because I had heard similar descriptions about surgeons and their teams from other non-medical friends and acquaintances before, and especially the argument that military-like leadership of a surgeon is needed, particularly in an operating theatre. However, in order to tease out an explanation I commented inquisitively.

"Surgeon – 'the commander with his crew', sounds like a military unit on a parade?"

"Precisely, and so it should be Mr M. You know I used to work in the army and I feel that a chain of command brings out the best from people as long as those who are in command lead well. I think that is very important in a surgical occupation where there should be no room for error. The surgeon I met today appeared to be the commander, I could feel that he commanded the respect of his team; so I know that my son is in safe hands."

Already aware about the tiered framework of the world of surgery the young trainee makes a quiet entry into it. Like a newly born cub inhaling the first breath in the wild, the junior tries to mingle with the pride, build relationships with fellow cubs, endure the aura and authority of the powerful members of the pride – both young and old, and starts by walking along quietly with the rest of the group. The individual follows the Kipling maxim that a man-cub is a man-cub and must learn all the laws of the jungle.

The *Oxford Dictionary* defines an apprentice as *a person who is learning a trade from a skilled employer, having agreed to work for a fixed period at low wages*. That is exactly what a surgical trainee used to be during my training years – low wages, long hours and an uncertain future. Even though the institution where you worked paid you, the real employer was the boss to whom you were accountable and responsible. It was imperative to remain in his or her good books. To begin with, the conversations with the boss used to be limited and generally one-sided. One had to learn to be a good listener and choose an opportune moment to speak when the chief was in a good mood, for instance after having performed a slick surgical operation. This continues to be the case in many countries even today.

In order to take care of each layer of authority separately the newcomer has to learn speedily about the likes and dislikes of each individual within the hierarchy.

Some of the commands end up at various nexuses along the

chain but some travel all the way down and terminate at the bottom of the chain at the weakest link – in the new apprentice's territory. A few of these can be unreasonable or even bizarre. Two separate first hand experiences by colleagues described below illustrate the point. In the second of the two anecdotes the message was brought home after a four-course meal.

THE PECKING ORDER (FROM DB, UK, 1984)

We used to go on a grand tour of the hospital at the end of each on-take day to see all surgical patients admitted under our care. The chief (who was the senior-most consultant), senior lecturer, lecturer, senior registrar, junior registrar, senior house officer, ward sister and I (house officer) were on this particular ward round. Being my first day I did not think that I had too much to worry about. But I was wrong.

The entourage arrived at the bedside of a charming little, blind and partially deaf but fit octogenarian lady who had been admitted during the previous night with vague abdominal pain. After a few questions to her the chief turned towards the senior lecturer and asked, "Has this lady had a rectal examination?"

The senior lecturer turned to the senior registrar and whispered the question,

"Did you examine her and did you perform a rectal?"

Without saying much but flashing his eyebrows the senior registrar looked anxiously at the registrar. Like a paper boat floating on a rapidly flowing undulating stream the question moved down the chain through tacit body language and stopped suddenly at me. At this point the ward sister looked at me, and with an aura of authority, in a very posh accent said loudly, "Did you undertake a rectal examination?"

As all eyes focussed on me I felt the weight of the world on my chest. My heart started galloping, and since I had nobody to pass on the question to, nervously I muttered the word: "No."

Like a fast moving electric signal my response travelled up the chain to the great man who then said, "Well! Somebody should do one."

Nothing was actually said but the orders were glanced down the escalator and stopped at me. So I had to go and get a pair of latex gloves, lubricating jelly etc. and perform a rectal examination to check for constipation and other abnormalities.

The ward sister explained to the lady what was going to happen. She was suitably positioned, and as I was about to commence the examination the sweet old soul spoke to me over her shoulder and said, "I am so pleased that you are getting to the bottom of my troubles, doctor."

CARRYING THE PUPPY (FROM MH, UK)

This was early nineteen eighties – my first posting as PRHO (pre registration house officer) in surgery at a large district general hospital. The head of the firm was a tight-lipped Englishman, very traditional and old fashioned, not far from the point of retirement. He loved tennis and apparently used to play the game as a youngster. He and his wife would invite his juniors for dinner at their home once every year in the month of June, on a Saturday during the course of Wimbledon tennis tournament.

The setting was gorgeous – the house was located in a leafy suburb outside London, which had a sizeable dining patio with a large, colourful back garden with beautifully laid and striped turf. The evening was truly formal – the table had been laid before our arrival and printed nametags directed us to our chairs. We had an enjoyable four-course meal and after finishing the dessert everyone started chatting relaxingly, when suddenly the old man announced, "Let us go for a walk, chaps."

Everyone got up and followed the boss. There was still some light in the horizon when we started the march. Interestingly, the invitees formed a line comprising the boss, followed by the senior registrar, registrar and senior house officers in that order. The last in the queue was I, who was also entrusted with an additional responsibility – to carry the boss's little puppy in my arms.

For the junior though, there are many other lessons to learn. As you get to know other personalities in the patch, with experience you become wise enough to distinguish friends from foes. With time the tenderfoot creates alliances and devises ways to deal with tricky situations and ward off impending dangers and conflicts, which can appear in different shapes and forms.

The friendly face (from MN, UK)

After qualifying from a medical school in Pakistan during the nineteen seventies and working there for a few years I immigrated to the UK in 1981. Before leaving my country I sought advice from my seniors who had returned after training in the UK, about the dos and don'ts of working in a UK hospital. Amongst other things I was advised to always carry in my white coat pocket a tourniquet, which was to be used to draw blood from patients for various laboratory tests.

On the first morning of my first posting as a senior house officer at a London hospital I arrived on the ward and was greeted by a locum registrar. Accompanied by a smart female staff nurse with conspicuously dark and big eyes, we went round and saw each patient on that ward. All of them were under care of the boss for whom I was going to work. Following that we went to see our other patients who were scattered on various wards all round the hospital. In all we must have seen a total of about forty patients. The registrar passed on to me instructions about each patient, which I noted meticulously in my pocket notebook. The rounds finished well after midday when he suddenly waved an abrupt good-bye and disappeared into the corridor crowd for lunch.

I went back to the main ward and took stock of the long list of things to do. That included taking blood samples from about twenty patients. The staff nurse who had accompanied us on the ward round earlier in the day welcomed me back. "If you need help with form filling give me a shout," she said with a friendly smile.

As I started bleeding the first patient she came near the foot end of the bed and said, "The laboratory takes routine blood samples only up to 2pm; specimens received thereafter are processed next day. Also I am not sure if you know that the boss will be going round tomorrow and he likes to see the latest blood results on all patients."

As if that wasn't enough, smilingly she piled another brick on my already burdened shoulder, "Also please do not forget about prescriptions for take home drugs for ward discharges." Thankfully my bleeper went off at this point and that interrupted her flow.

I continued to receive calls every few minutes from other wards regarding patient discharge certificates and other requests. However, I carried on diligently with my task of taking blood samples from one patient after another, while the demands from other quarters became louder and more frequent. The pressure on me intensified. By then I did not know where I was and in the process I lost my tourniquet – probably I had thrown it in the yellow sharps box with blood-soiled syringes. Since it was my first working day in a new country I didn't know what to do, but I went to my friendly staff nurse and asked meekly, "Do you have a tourniquet on the ward?"

"No, doctors bring their own but you can use a urinary catheter instead," she said with a grin on her face.

"That was helpful advice," I thought to myself. "A catheter can be tied around the patient's upper arm or wrist and can work as a tourniquet." So I rushed to the utility room, picked a blue coloured sterile urinary catheter – one I had never seen before. I unpacked it from its package, and without wasting any time went back to my business. About half an hour later the friendly staff nurse came again, this time informing me that the ward sister wanted to see me urgently in her office.

"Why?" I asked.

With a frown and with her eyes wide open she warned me, "She will tell you. By the way, she does not mince her words."

Apprehensively I went into Sister J's office, where a middle aged, elegant looking lady in a dark blue uniform with an ambience around her was standing. She pointed me to the vacant chair and no sooner I sat down she started authoritatively, "Where did you get the silicone catheter from?"

Oh! That is what a silicone catheter is – the blue catheter that I was using, I thought to myself as I sat in the chair uneasily. But I had nothing to hide, so I said, "I got it from the utility room."

"Did you seek permission doctor, and by the way where is your own tourniquet?" By now the pressure on me was unbearable.

"I am sorry sister, I should have asked. I lost my tourniquet somewhere."

"Do you know how expensive a silicone catheter is compared to an ordinary catheter?"

In all honesty I did not – I did not even know the difference between the two. I had never seen a silicone urinary catheter before. Therefore I decided not to answer.

"Ten times the price of a latex catheter. And you used the last size sixteen that I had in stock." The hammering continued.

Finally she concluded by saying, "I will write to the medical staffing department and ask them to deduct the cost of the catheter from your wages."

I simply wished to leave the room and was relieved to hear the words, "You can go now."

The day was long and tedious and as I started walking back to my hostel room I was having serious reservations about whether to carry on with my surgical pursuits in the UK.

A couple of months later during the Christmas party, Sister J and I started chatting. By then we knew each other better and were on friendlier terms. During the course of the conversation I asked her, "By the way, who told you about the silicone catheter that I used as a tourniquet?"

Guess what? It was my friendly big-eyed staff nurse!

A NARROW ESCAPE (FROM IK, UK)

I worked as a locum senior house officer in a busy surgical department at a hospital in London during the 1980s. On Friday afternoons my job was to assess patients who were due to be admitted for major surgery during the week after, take their blood samples and send these to the laboratory for analysis. It was essentially the infantile version of present day pre-assessment clinic.

I was due to work for the first time in that clinic in the afternoon and earlier in the day my registrar warned me about what to expect, "Do not forget to meet the sister in-charge before you start the clinic this afternoon. She is a diamond but can sometimes be rough at the edges."

As directed, I arrived early and went straight to sister's office. She was an oblong looking figure, short and stocky – but stern looking, in her late fifties. Seated in a small round chair she looked like a boiled egg that had been placed neatly on an eggcup. As I entered she inspected me in a flash from head to foot through her small-framed glasses. As I introduced myself she got up abruptly from her chair and took me on a mini-tour of her dominion, finally showing me a room full of syringes, bottles, dressings and an examination couch.

"You will take bloods here and remember, no mess, Doctor, do you understand? If you create a mess you will not come here again," she concluded firmly.

Minutes after leaving the room she returned and delivered a postscript warning, "And don't ask my staff to clean up the mess. You will have to clean it yourself."

I resented her manner but had to put up and without showing any emotion muttered, "Yes, sister."

Whilst I was still thinking in my subconscious mind about her attitude and her one-way conversation with me, I began seeing the first patient, Mr S. After examining him and completing the notes I got ready to take a blood sample from him for various tests. As I withdrew blood from him into a 20ml syringe, for a second or so I lost my concentration, the syringe overfilled and its entire content dripped on the floor and the syringe parted company from the needle. With the tourniquet still on the patient's arm further blood dripped away – on the couch, floor, patient's clothes, my hands and white coat – practically everywhere; the room was painted spotty red.

"Sorry, Mr S…" I said sheepishly after removing the tourniquet . "What am I going to do if she finds out?" I muttered involuntarily, to which he responded with, "Pardon!"

Mr S had no idea about my state of panic as he tried to cheer me up. "Don't worry Doctor, I donate blood regularly. You can take another syringe of blood."

I stood still for a minute or so and then sneaked outside the room. Fortunately I found a junior nurse in her mid-twenties busily writing notes. I approached her cautiously and said, "Can you help me with a patient please? He is on the couch."

As she came into the room, she gasped, "Oh, dear, what a horrible mess! You are in a hell of a trouble; if she sees this, she will kill you – and me too, if she sees me here."

Mr S appeared rather bewildered but stayed calm as I closed the door quietly.

Amidst a shower of apologies to him, we (junior nurse and I) – with some help from Mr S, managed to wipe everything clean, hide the mess in a yellow bag and a sharps bin, change the sheet, rub the floor and trolley clean, sponge the patient, draw a fresh blood sample, label the bottles and rewrite the forms. There was of course the constant fear of sister appearing suddenly at the door.

As I opened the door after the job was done, my nursing colleague who was going off duty sneaked away quietly on a tiptoe with the words, "Nice to have met you, good luck."

Phew! That was a narrow escape from the jaws of danger!

DOUBLE TROUBLE (FROM HH, UK)

The story dates back thirty years during my tenure as senior house officer in a two-consultant urology department. One of our bosses was keen that any patients with a permanent or short term urinary catheter for bladder drainage had the catheter strapped to their thigh by a special technique, which was apparently his very own brainchild, and which the trainee had to learn during the first week of posting in the department. "These old boys get confused in the dark and pull their catheters – this technique prevents injury." He would repeat the commandment every few weeks.

The other and younger of the two consultants was a vehement opponent of strapping to the point of getting upset if he saw a catheter strapped to the thigh on any of his patients. "You know this strapping business is simply a grandmother's tale, I never strap my patients' catheters and never had a problem." He would remind everyone emphatically from time to time.

We trainees had learnt to cope with the situation and adhered to these directives as far as possible. However, if we sensed that there was a danger of being caught breaking the laws of respective charters, we had a novel trick up our sleeve that we used – albeit in emergency situations only.

The anti-strapper went round on a Tuesday and the strapper on a Thursday. About ten minutes before their respective ward rounds we checked every bed and depending on whether it was a Tuesday or a Thursday, simply changed the name-plate of the boss at the head end of the bed, making sure that the name-plate matched with whether the catheter was strapped or not. The kings were happy and so were the subjects, but we knew that the trick was applicable only to newly admitted patients whom the bosses would not be able to recognise. During my one-year stay on that unit the tactic never failed.

Apprenticeship may have challenges but there are rewards too. Triumphs, however small, work like water and sunshine for the trainee. A well accomplished piece of work, spotting a clinical sign, making a correct diagnosis, cutting the end of a stitch neatly, being thanked for being a good assistant, listening to a compliment from a patient, a commending remark by the boss or other inhabitants of the territory, seeing one's name printed in a journal – anything that lifts the spirits makes the day worthwhile. Rewards can come in other forms too.

I was working as a senior resident at a teaching hospital in India during the late 1970s. This was before the era of keyhole surgery. Mr P, the patient on the operation table, was a grossly overweight, high-ranking government official on whom the boss was about to make an incision. The target was a 15mm stone stuck in the lower third of ureter (the tube connecting the kidney to bladder), causing backpressure effects on his kidney. That day everyone in theatre was unusually business-like – no jokes from the boss, no chitchat with the anaesthetist and no discussion about cricket scores; the whole atmosphere appeared grim.

I had started in the firm a couple of weeks before and was still not fully acclimatised to the environmental temperature and hierarchical structure of the department. Prudency demanded that I remained quiet and observant.

I was the second assistant and was commanded to stand on the surgeon's side of the table (patient's right side), on the surgeon's left side. Soon we were inside the patient's abdomen. The boss arranged the retractors to give him wide access. I was ordered to hold one of the broad retractors with two hands to create a wide space and make the chief's' job easier.

The boss started looking for the ureter using his hands and instruments. My senior colleague who was the first assistant and I tried our best to help by pulling harder and harder on the retractors, but the ureter could not be located. After a while he repositioned the retractors and launched another search, using all tricks of the trade that he knew, but after two hours' hunt the ureter remained elusive. With each passing minute the boss was becoming more frustrated and edgy. As is usual in such a situation the assistants started feeling the heat.

The retractors were rearranged once again, and while my retractor was moved, my fingers could sense something like a stone touching the retractor edge. However, in view of the tense situation all round I decided to keep quiet. Further attempts by the boss were unproductive and at that point he moved away from the table to check the X-rays, which were suspended in the viewing box on one of the theatre walls. The stone was clearly visible on the X-ray.

During that interval I discreetly put my hand into the wound and could clearly feel a stone like object. With hindsight I feel that the ureter and the stone within it were being pulled away from the centre of the wound by my retractor and that was probably the reason why the boss was facing the difficulty. On his return to the table I plucked up the courage to speak and articulated nervously, "Sir, I can feel the stone."

No one responded to my comment; the first assistant glanced at me rather disapprovingly – telling me to mind my own business by furrowing his bushy eyebrows. There was silence for a few minutes after which the boss turned to me suddenly and said, "Did you say you felt the stone?"

"Yes sir, I did."

Turning his face towards me he enquired. "Are you sure?"

"Well, I think so…" I responded hesitatingly.

"In that case we will be your assistants and you try to get the stone out," he commanded.

Now it was my turn to feel edgy, but I had no choice. I put my hand into the wound and could feel the stone again, which infused me with confidence. I repositioned the retractors, held the ureter and the stone within a special clamp, incised the ureter and, like a magician pulling a handkerchief from an empty bottle, delivered the stone. There was applause all round. Without saying much the boss left soon after. The first assistant and I completed the rest of the operation. That was one of the happiest days of my life and as the news about my feat spread amongst my colleagues I felt elated for a few days.

Three days later the boss asked me to follow him to the room where Mr P was admitted. Mr P looked cheerful; his family were with him when we arrived. After exchange of pleasantries the boss began by saying, "Mr P, you should be grateful to this man who came to our rescue. He removed your stone after I struggled for about two hours."

I felt embarrassed and did not know what to say.

A few weeks later the boss called me again, this time to his office and said, "I appreciate your help during Mr P's surgical procedure and would like to invite you for a meal; my wife and I will meet you at the K's Restaurant on Saturday at 8pm. Is that okay with you?

"Yes sir, I will be there," I mumbled unbelievingly.

And we went for a meal together – the boss, his wife and I. We enjoyed a three-course dinner followed by ice cream at a favourite spot in town. During the whole evening we discussed a number of topics ranging from politics to sports but did not talk about work or the patient. At the end the great man said, "… thank you for getting me out of a deep hole."

Apprenticeship in surgery involves practical training under supervision that is appropriate to the level of seniority and surgical competence of the trainee. Keen to learn and imbibe as many tricks of the trade from as many people as possible, a working day is never the same for a trainee. Eager to test the surgical waters the trainee is on the look out for opportunities all the time. These can appear suddenly and need to be grabbed with both hands whenever possible.

WIN-WIN FOR ALL (FROM TS, INDIA, 1996)

Much like a football or a rugby captain some bosses have a habit of huddling together with their team before starting the day in theatre, so that everyone knows who is operating on which patient and who is assisting. Some go through this exercise the day before the operation day. Like a charity distribution centre, trainees expect that they would get some of the pickings and prizes, and be allowed to undertake procedures independently. That also gives trainees an indication of what the boss thinks about their level of competence.

Prof S used to summon his team to his office on a Wednesday evening to distribute responsibilities for the all-day list next day. One of the senior residents (Dr T) could not believe his ears when the professor said to him, "You are going to do this nephrectomy (removal of kidney) and Dr P is going to assist you. If you need any more help, let me know, but read it up thoroughly tonight."

"Yes sir," he replied excitedly.

Next day, looking quietly confident, Dr T arrived in theatre all geared up to undertake the major procedure. As he came in, the theatre sister stopped him and said, "Nephrectomy will have to be cancelled. There is no blood available for transfusion – the relative who was supposed to donate was found to be unfit."

"What?" replied Dr T in disbelief; and after a pause he added, "Please do not cancel the case, I will see what I can do." And suddenly he disappeared from the scene and reappeared after about an hour.

"Sister, there is blood available for the nephrectomy patient. Can we please carry on with the list as planned?"

Dr T performed the nephrectomy without any problems whatsoever. At the end of the procedure the theatre sister commented, "Very well done – we did not need blood after all!"

"I know but some other patient will benefit from the pint of blood that I donated this morning," he replied with a broad smile.

"Did you really? Well! I suppose it's a win-win for all, someone will benefit from the blood you donated and you got your reward – your first nephrectomy."

All surgeons would have a story to tell about an embarrassing moment they witnessed, or were personally involved with, during the course of their training. Most of these are of a minor nature but some can become serious enough to create discomforting situations and land the junior in difficulty.

PAINTING IN BLACK (FROM HW, 1992)

Long before the introduction of 'Informed Consent' in the UK, I worked for a few days as a locum house officer in a surgical unit in London. On my last day in the post my registrar asked me to clerk a patient who was admitted to have surgery on the following day for a large hydrocele (fluid collection in the scrotal sac). He also instructed me to mark the correct side of surgery and get the patient to sign a consent form.

After completing the patient's notes and getting him to sign the form (which was only a formality in those days) I got hold of an indelible black marker pen. Having never marked a patient previously I was unsure of what to do next. I did wonder though, how anyone could get the side wrong with an enormous swelling like that. Nevertheless, I had to carry out my line manager's orders.

With no seniors around to ask, like an expert painter I proceeded to colour the scrotal skin black over the enormous hydrocele with my indelible marker making sure that every bit of skin over the swelling was painted. The elderly patient obligingly let me finish the job and thanked me profusely.

Later that afternoon the ward sister bleeped me urgently. As I arrived on the scene I found her in a frantic state. "How did Mr S end up with half of the scrotum looking black?" she asked.

I had no other option but to confess and explain to her what had happened. She didn't say much but gave me a stern look as we walked together to the patient's bed. Nervously I offered the gentleman my meek explanation along with profuse apologies. He laughed loudly which made me more nervous as he was led away to the bathroom by one of the junior nurses for a scrub.

My locum job at the hospital ended the same evening but he must have undergone hydrocele repair the following day.

I remember the incident every time I mark a patient prior to surgery.

THINK BEFORE YOU SPEAK (FROM DM, UK, *1988*)

It was my second day as a house officer on the surgical firm. I accompanied my senior house officer to see a lady in her thirties who had attended the Emergency Department on her own complaining of lower abdominal pain. She was lying on a couch in one of the cubicles.

My senior colleague took a detailed history and examined her in the presence of a student nurse and me, following which he organised blood and urine tests, including a pregnancy test.

However, without any further explanation to the patient he left the cubicle and I followed him, which meant that the lady was in the cubicle with the student nurse.

The lady's husband had apparently been away on overseas business for three months and by sheer co-incidence had arrived back in the country on the same day. When he reached home and heard about his wife's illness he rushed straight to the hospital and joined his wife in the cubicle, soon after we had left.

On our return to the cubicle we found the lady sitting with her husband; his travel luggage was tugged in one corner. Without a second thought my senior colleague said to the lady, "Congratulations, you are pregnant. We will send you to EPAC (early pregnancy assessment clinic) for evaluation."

That was a big mistake – the announcement was a rude shock to the couple. After an initial period of silence there was pandemonium; the patient started crying and the husband became angry and abusive. He stormed out and the lady became abusive towards the senior house officer. In a state of hysterical anger she volunteered the information that not only had the husband been away for three months but also that he had undergone vasectomy two years before.

The senior house officer was devastated but couldn't do much except offer regrets and apologies. For me that was a lesson about confidentiality.

A MUDDY MESS (FROM DB, UK)

During the mid-1980s I was working as a surgical registrar at a hospital in southeast England. One of the pleasures of working there was the close proximity of the hospital to the local rugby club. I had just finished playing when I got an urgent call from the Emergency Department. I jumped over the fence and presented myself at the department that was only fifty yards away from the rugby pitch. There I was asked to see a young male motorcyclist who had been involved in a road accident.

Examination by the Emergency Department staff had indicated blood and fluid in the abdominal cavity, probably signifying a ruptured internal organ – very likely the spleen. However, he was clinically stable with a normal blood pressure. I advised the patient that he might need an urgent laparotomy (exploration of abdomen) under general anaesthetic. The patient looked at me in horror and said, "I hope you will have a wash first, won't you Doc?" I suddenly realised that I was still in my rugby kit.

I was ashamed and apologised. Needless to add, I did have a thorough wash and operated on the young man, and he made an uneventful recovery.

A HAPPY DOG (FROM RB)

In Scotland during the 1960s, private hospitals were quite small with very few laboratory facilities. At one particular hospital, after any operation, the removed organ or tissue would be taken to the main NHS hospital, which was a couple of miles away, for examination by the histo-pathologist.

On this occasion a male patient underwent open operation for removal of prostate gland on a Saturday morning. The female surgical registrar who assisted the boss with the operation was entrusted with the responsibility of transporting the excised prostate gland to the NHS hospital.

Several weeks later, after finishing the ward round, the boss asked the registrar, "By the way I did not see the histology report on the prostate gland we removed at the private hospital a few weeks ago."

The registrar blushed and was speechless for a few moments and then replied nervously, "Sir, I hoped you would never ask but I must make a confession. I wrapped the prostate gland in a newspaper and put it on the back seat of my car. Because it was a Saturday morning I had the family dog in the back of the car. On my way to the hospital I stopped at the local grocery store. Unfortunately while I was there the dog ate the prostate gland! Sir, I am really very sorry."

The boss walked away in disgust.

Funny but ashamedly true – that is how one would characterise the last story, but that was the surgical world during the 1960s.

I had my embarrassing moments too during my training years. One of these was when I was working as a senior resident in a tertiary care hospital in India during the late seventies. This was a large department and in such units it is not uncommon to have several trainees or assistants of a similar cadre, like three residents, two registrars or two assistant professors and so on. Much like a group of school children there is a sense of dormant competition amongst the equals, with everyone trying to be in the good books of the chief.

Our professor was a gem of a gentleman and was widely respected for his simplicity and straightforwardness. He admired juniors who were brief and to the point because he himself was a man of precision. There were four senior residents in the department including me, and all of us used to get ready for the professorial ward round on Thursday mornings. That was the highlight of the weekly timetable. We put in special effort to know the clinical details of every admitted patient, just in case a question was asked. In the event of a question or a comment being fired into the air without a clear target, much like a group of kindergarten children, sometimes all of us would jump with an answer – often together.

One Thursday, in the middle of the ward round we came to a male patient who had been admitted in the small hours of the morning with inability to pass urine. None of us had seen him at the time of admission. We started hiding behind one another to avoid eye contact with the professor, who was intelligent enough to realise our predicament. Without making any further enquiries he started asking the patient directly about his problems. Following that he moved round to the right side of the bed and asked the patient to expose the abdomen and the genital area.

The moment the patient rolled down the sheet and his underclothes and exposed his external genitals, like a silly bunch of jokers all four of us piped up in a disorderly chorus: "Err! I know him... actually... yes, I remember – err, yes – but... sir..."

The patient had distinctive areas of leucoderma (white patches on the skin) on the penis and scrotum by which we all recognised him instantly. Prior to this admission he had attended our department many times and each of us had performed urethral dilatation (stretching of water passage using special curved metallic rods called bougies) on him in the past. We all had registered his features down under but none of us could remember his face. The episode left all of us red-faced with embarrassment.

Despite its triumphs and tribulations residency is the foundation on which the surgical structure stands. With time the trainee learns to run with the fast and the furious and slow down with the sure and the steady; grabs opportunities as they arise during long nights spent between theatres and wards amidst mugs of tea and coffee, and acquires the insight to tread carefully along tortuous territories. As in every walk of life emotional perks nurture the wellbeing and development of the apprentice. A word of praise from others and the fatigue is all gone. A neatly accomplished piece of work gives the junior a sleepless night and so does a patient who develops a post-operative complication. Every step, however, small or big is a memory; and every tumble is a memory too. You remember the first appendix, or the first gall bladder you removed – or the first stone you fished out successfully. You also recall situations where you had to seek help to bail you out.

I have heard a number of synonyms used for a trainee/resident:

dogsbody, slave, robot, walking dead and so on. In my own experience and from what I have heard from others, despite the long hours and caffeine overdose, residency/training is the most enjoyable period of one's surgical career. Like a toddler a trainee learns to roll over, sit up, wobble through the first step, walk with eyes fixed on the ground, trot with care, venture to run and finally gain adulthood and gallop away.

4

THE TRANSITION

The end of residency signals metamorphosis of the individual from an adolescent to an adult. The trainee is awarded a certificate by peers and elders that bears testimony of having acquired the capability to care for and if necessary make cuts on fellow humans without supervision. The surgical training may be over, but apprenticeship is not. That is a life-long process, which has no end point. There is a lesson to learn everyday – technical, clinical, moral, emotional, ethical, psychological and more. That is because technology and science are constantly on the move. Moreover, patients are living entities – diverse from one another. The same surgical procedure performed on two different patients is never exactly the same.

The occasion that every trainee dreams of, and every clinician remembers with a sense of fondness and fulfilment is the day of being appointed as a consultant or a faculty member. The decision to crown the newcomer is taken by the elder statesmen and stateswomen of the territory in closed alleyways of power. The candidate may have come to the end of the residency but due to factors such as lack of confidence, wrong career choice or inadequate and/or insufficient training, may still need support. Yet the person may be an excellent work colleague with a great temperament. Conversely, the individual may be a skilled craftsman and/or a high class diagnostician but an awful personality to work with. The selectors are entrusted with the task of analysing the strengths and weaknesses of applicants in a short space of time, assess their skills, knowledge and temperament, identify the unfinished, inept or unsuitable end product, and judge how well the new appointee would fit within the organisation and *vice versa*. Once appointed the deed is done – a good appointment builds and a bad one wrecks a department or an organisation. There is a lot of truth in the statement: you can divorce your spouse but you can never get rid of the colleague you have just appointed.

Having sat on tens of consultant interview panels I know that it is not an easy exercise. CVs, interview performances and references are not the only criteria on which a judgment is made – a number of other factors come into play on the day. Sometimes it is difficult to perceive the boundary where confidence ends and arrogance and recklessness begins. That is particularly important when you are making a surgical appointment. The following anecdote about the deliberations of a consultant appointment panel that I sat on, illustrates the point.

The appointments panel comprised the CEO, three clinician-managers from within the organisation and two external assessors, who were both clinicians. An experienced non-executive director was chairing the meeting. There were three prospective candidates for one consultant surgeon appointment. After the interviews were concluded the committee chairman opened the discussion that went something like as follows.

"Ladies and gentlemen, I want to know from each of you, your first, second and third preferences with a two minute summary about the reasons for your choices."

After the individual summary presentations it was clear that there were two candidates to choose from; but each of the two candidates had managed to secure three out of the total of six votes.

"Well, would anyone reconsider after hearing that result?" asked the chairman.

All the six panel members replied in negative.

"I want to ask the three of you who are in favour of appointing candidate A the most important reason for not appointing candidate B?"

All three gave the same reasons in different words: "He appeared too boastful and arrogant. He wouldn't let me even finish the question," said the first panel member.

"Did you not see how he sat in the chair, with his right leg over the left knee with the right foot pointing up, and the way he talked? Frankly, that was quite irritating." That was the opinion of the second member. "It was all about me, me and me, honestly I feel he will be bad news for the department and the organisation," concluded the third member.

The chairman then addressed the other three panel members, "Now I want to ask the three of you who prefer candidate B the most important reasons for your decision?"

The respective answers from three panel members were similar but were worded differently.

"I felt that he is a confident chap, really sure of himself." "This man will push the department in the right direction. He has the oomph and the go." "He might be pushy but what do you expect from a young man at this stage of his life?"

The chairman then asked the three supporters of candidate A the reasons for their decision. Respectively they described him as 'amiable', 'gentlemanly' and 'well mannered'. The three opponents judged him as 'slow', 'timid' and 'sluggish'.

It was an extraordinary experience for me to witness the proceedings, wherein the same person, giving the same performance, registered two contrasting images in two different mirrors. A debate followed during which I argued for the confident (arrogant?) i.e. candidate B. The matter was ultimately settled with the chairman's vote. He sided with the departmental head; who was a firm supporter of candidate B.

Notwithstanding my arguments in favour of the appointed candidate during the panel deliberations, after leaving the committee room I felt uneasy for the rest of the day. "Did I make the right judgement?" I was asking myself. "Only time will tell who was right and who was wrong?" I pondered.

Like a young and agile bird venturing on test flights that become longer and longer with each trip, the new recruit plunges into the wild to travel the tiger country. The leap into adulthood is a challenge for the new appointee and generates a bundle of emotions – ambitious excitement mixed with determination and a feeling of freedom and independence. Yet deep down lurks the thought of a heavy weight of responsibility. The youngster's behaviour can range from: because I said so to let's get a second opinion for every problem, big or small. Generally, the individual who admits to shortcomings in training and the need for further development is preferable to the one who compensates inexperience by being boastful.

The new kid in town is the subject of off-the-cuff conversations amongst colleagues and staff members. Comments are made and judgements pronounced.

One of the ancient looking surgeons strolls lazily into the surgeons' changing room and on seeing another old timer fires the question, "How is the new orthopod doing, old chap?"

"Very slick – will go a long way – good lad and a nice fella too!"

Holding a well filled bread roll in her right hand and a bottle of coke in the left, a young and bubbly scrub nurse rushes into the theatre sitting room and makes a statement, "I am starving (nibble) – it took us three hours (nibble-nibble); what a pain! Can you believe it, the new guy whatever his name is, took nearly an hour just to drape the patient (nibble-nibble) – Mr Z would have whipped the whole thing out in twenty minutes."

A larger than life anaesthetist in extra-large theatre blues with tension oozing from his scarlet cheeks and ears strolls up and down the theatre corridor and announces to a colleague, "Tell you what, I have rung my wife to cancel the evening. We won't finish in time. It took us two hours to position the patient – a little to the right, now a little to the left – made everyone sweat! Dear-o-dear, this new chap seems to be in love with himself, strokes himself all the time – I mean his face and hair; I am going to give him a pair of mirrors for Christmas and tell them to fix these to two sides of the operating table."

An ODA (operation department assistant) with many theatre miles on his clock – on his lunch break, seemingly absorbed in his tabloid newspaper whilst simultaneously munching on a large chunk of homemade sandwich, suddenly explodes and throws a remark at everyone present, "Where do they bring such jokers from? They should first give them induction lessons on proper behaviour. Spoiled my day, there are still shenanigans going on in that theatre."

An evenly shaped, delicate looking senior sister, who appears to be enjoying her break and the cup a soup, addresses a senior surgeon who is seated at the other end of the room and is absorbed with a pile of paperwork that his secretary brought for him to look at: "And by the way Mr M, I was with the new general surgery bloke last week. You did well to pick him – what a nice chap – a true gentleman, came in, smiled at everyone, finished the job – neat and tidy – off and away."

The new recruits can also sense that they are being observed or talked about. Gestures, body language and casual remarks – good and bad – from onlookers, assistants and passers-by, many of which are casual and unintentional, can create as well as ease pressure on the newcomer. The novice has to learn other lessons too, like not crossing the path of a ruling lord of the jungle – a lesson that ruined a day of my life during the late 1980s.

This was my second week and my first theatre list as a locum consultant at this UK hospital. I was about to start a surgical procedure on a septuagenarian man when I asked the scrub nurse,

"Do you have a piano diathermy pedal which has both coagulation and cutting knobs together rather than separately?"

"Yes, we have one in the other theatre." And she asked one of the circulation nurses to bring a piano pedal from the other theatre.

After finishing the procedure I left my theatre and as I started walking up the long theatre corridor on my way to surgeons' sitting room, I saw a man in his late fifties, in theatre greens with half moon glasses hooked on the tip of his nose, walking restlessly in the opposite direction. He stopped abruptly right in front of me, blocked my path and said, "Are you the locum who was operating in Theatre 4?"

"Yes, I am."

"How dare you take the piano pedal from my theatre?"

As I looked at him I could see the blush on his round and chubby face, and raw anger exuding from his eyes. But I kept my composure and replied, "I did not take it. I asked the theatre staff who got it for me from somewhere."

Pointing his right index finger at me he retorted, "Don't you ever dare to touch any of the gadgets without asking me; is that clear?" And with that he removed his glasses and walked back briskly.

The suddenness and rudeness of the episode made me numb and dumb. It was like one of the Laurel and Hardy episodes with powerless Laurel being disparaged by pompous Hardy for something he was not directly responsible. Helplessly I watched him pace back up the corridor until he disappeared into his theatre. I walked slowly to the surgeon's room and sank into a chair. A little while later the scrub nurse who had assisted me sat in the chair beside me and said, "Sorry Mr M, that was my fault. I heard he gave you a hard time. You have to realise that he is the big boss who rules this place. No one ever dares to cross him."

I chose not to reply but it took me couple of days to wipe off the incident from my troubled mind.

Jungle creatures, corridor gossipers and in-house opinion makers do count, but the most important people who ultimately matter are patients and their families whose lives are touched one way or the other by the new broom. In most cases, however, it is the word of mouth that determines a surgeon's reputation. A skilful surgeon with bad mannerism is tolerated for a while and an individual with substandard surgical ability but with great personal touch gets into difficulty eventually. To possess all qualities is an asset.

It is no surprise that after years of toil the end product becomes an amalgam of trade tricks and influences from a range of people – bosses, colleagues and peers – senior and junior, and even patients. It is not only surgical tips and techniques that are perfected but like a growing child the individual imbibes habits, body language, mannerism, posture, ticks and movements and much more. Even words – some good and some not so good, get tethered to the new incumbent and bounce off from time to time, which work colleagues, patients, and families at the new place of work find difficult to comprehend, at least to begin with. Here are a few phrases that I have heard over the years.

Declaring a patient unfit for a surgical operation: "He is not fit even for a haircut."

Describing the operative findings after undertaking abdominal surgery on a patient: "The liver looked really beaten up."

Describing a patient with no urinary output after a road traffic accident: "His beans have sustained a nasty whack. Let's hope they wake up."

Whilst looking through an endoscope up the ureter (the tube connecting the kidney to urinary bladder), with a good view of the ureteric lumen: "This ureter looks like a motorway."

Boasting to a medical colleague after repairing a ruptured abdominal aortic aneurysm: "I was fixing a burst balloon."

Swaggering to a resident just before starting the surgical procedure on a patient with large piles, "I don't know why they all come to me? Look at these – these are massive, they look like cauliflowers!"

Speaking to a manager on the phone after finishing an operation successfully where there was excessive bleeding: "Can you please ring me later, I have been in red up to my gills."

Surgeons also use catchphrases and invented expressions, probably to feel good about themselves and to impress others, and possibly to make others pause and ponder. However, coded words and phrases can be a source of confusion and can even lead to a state of panic. A theatre manager recounts an interesting incident of her career.

SAY WHAT YOU MEAN! (FROM KW, UK)

The incident happened more than twenty-five years ago during my first week as a qualified registered nurse. In those days it was considered rude to interrupt surgeons during an operation and very few people dared to ask a question. All their commands had to be carried out. I was assigned the responsibility of a circulating nurse for the first case. The patient was a lady undergoing open nephrectomy (removal of kidney). By coincidence this was also the second month for the newly appointed consultant surgeon, Mr B. The scrub nurse was also relatively junior in cadre and experience, but had worked in theatres for about two years.

The procedure was progressing smoothly but soon after opening the abdomen the surgeon said, "A peanut please?" The scrub nurse looked at me inquisitively. I shrugged my shoulders and signalled that I didn't know what a peanut was. Whilst my nursing colleague and I were conversing with each other in sign language to try to decipher the meaning of a peanut, Mr B – who was engrossed with the job in hand, came out with another demand, "Can I have the magic stuff please?"

Once again the scrub nurse looked at me for help, but

I couldn't offer any. Meanwhile, Mr B who was still deeply involved with his work, repeated, "Can I have the magic stuff please?"

We both felt helpless and whisperingly I asked the anaesthetist if he knew what peanut and magic stuff were but he was not of much assistance either. I rushed to the theatre staff room and asked the nurses and doctors sitting there, "The new surgeon in Theatre 2 is asking for a peanut and the magic stuff. Does anyone know what these are?" One of the senior sisters immediately replied, "Mr G used to call a Lahey's swab – round pea shaped cotton ball – a peanut, but I don't know what magic stuff is."

Soon the larger than life sister-in-charge arrived on the scene and on hearing the story barged straight into theatre, "Young man, please say what you mean. What do you mean by a peanut, and for God's sake what is this magic stuff?" She enquired authoritatively in a deep Irish accent.

Mr B was suddenly disarmed. "Sorry Sister, I should have explained. Lahey's swab is pea shaped, that is why it used to be called a peanut at my previous place of work, and one of my ex-bosses used to call an absorbable haemostatic pack the magic stuff."

"And why was that so?" she demanded an explanation.

"Because the pack stops bleeding on contact with a bleeding surface and works like magic, I guess!" he replied.

"How interesting!" The senior sister then turned to us and said, "Girls, never be scared to ask the surgeon what he means. Sometimes they don't mean what they say, and at other times they don't say what they mean."

All new players are keen to stamp their authority on the newly acquired territory with prevalent usage of the pronoun 'I' in various conversations, in some cases to the point of annoyance to others, as in in the following example recounted by a senior anaesthetic colleague.

Who is taking the risk? (from *BJ, UK, 2000*)

The incident happened at a hospital in southeast England where I had worked as a consultant anaesthetist for about twenty years. That afternoon I was scheduled to work in day surgery theatre. One of the patients on the theatre list was a fifty years old, twenty stones, insulin-dependent diabetic man scheduled to have repair of a large uncomplicated inguinal hernia. After examining the patient on the day ward I said to him, "In my view it is unsafe for you to have the operation as a day case. I will have a chat about that with your surgeon."

A few minutes later the recently appointed surgeon Mr S – a well built but short-statured man in his late thirties who appeared to have a halo of arrogance around him, arrived on the scene. I had heard of him but had not met him in person before.

I approached him courteously and said, "Mr S, I am Dr G – your anaesthetist for this afternoon. I have examined all patients scheduled on your list and I feel that we should cancel the operation on the diabetic gentleman listed for hernia repair."

"Why?" He asked with a fixed expression on his face.

"Because he is an insulin-dependent diabetic, is grossly overweight and it's not an emergency."

"So?" replied Mr S snappily.

"In my view he is a high risk candidate for anaesthetic and surgery, I feel he is unfit to be done as a day case and his diabetes needs to be controlled first."

However, Mr S wouldn't agree with my assessment that the operation should be rescheduled and done as an in-patient. The conversation started transforming into a noisy argument, which was easily heard by all patients in the bay. "I will not be responsible if there are problems. I am warning you about the risks," I pleaded.

"He is my patient. You don't have to take the risk. I will take the risk," he retorted back.

At this point the patient got up from his bed, stood in

front of both of us and exploded, "Hold on a second, guys; can I remind you that it is not you who is taking the risk. I am the one taking the risk here. I am going home." And with that he picked up his belongings and left the ward.

For the newcomer there are other means to impress too – like charm and good mannerism but some use slang to seek attention. A colleague would use phrases such as: "Using Penicillin in this situation will be like pissing in the wind." – (meaning that the drug would not work), to a good effect. The expression generated a giggle amongst the audience and that boosted the individual's ego, which was reflected by his contented look and radiant smile.

A surgical colleague recalls his experience of working for a newly appointed surgical consultant. Every time the newcomer undertook a surgical procedure, he would ask his assistant, "That was a *pucca* job, wasn't it?" He wouldn't stop until the assistant replied, "Yes, it was." The reply worked like yeast for the dough and made him happy. That reminds me of an episode from my apprenticeship years that made someone happy.

After working in the UK for a number of years Dr D joined our department as a faculty member at the teaching hospital in Kashmir. He was excellent in his work. All residents including me – then at the bottom of the ladder, admired and respected his abilities as a surgeon and a teacher. Besides, he had fantastic bedside manners. I parted company with that unit a few months after his arrival.

A couple of years later I was working as a resident at another hospital in India hundreds of miles away. A young surgeon (Dr S) joined the unit as a faculty member. His background was similar to that of Dr D – FRCS and work experience in England. During an informal chat with Dr S, I mentioned about Dr D and his all round abilities, in particular his outstanding skills as a surgeon.

A few weeks later, I was assisting Dr S with a major emergency abdominal operation. The procedure went very well with no untoward hitches or complications. After finishing the procedure he and I went for a cup of tea in the hospital canteen, when out of the blue Dr S asked me, "Did you enjoy the operation?"

"Yes sir, I did."

"Did you like my operating technique?"

My truthful reply was, "Yes sir, I did."

And like a school kid he splashed out the crunch question, which I guess he had been itching to ask, "As much as you liked Dr D's work in your previous hospital?"

I managed a judicious reply that made his day.

Having withstood and survived the assessment by peers and colleagues – junior and senior, staff and patients – the newcomer finally settles into a rhythm. Over a period of time the youngster explores the high peaks and low troughs of the surgical landscape. Navigating repeatedly across its tantalising tributaries through smelly passages and bright red cesspools, every new day brings in new lessons. With the passage of time the fledgling surgeon grows in confidence, becomes more adept in technique, and with each new lesson feels self-assured to take on any challenge.

5

THE AURA

As days slip into weeks, weeks roll into months, and months add up to years, the surgical clock ticks on, and with each added mile the young adult grows in stature. Years of experience transform into wisdom and good judgment and the clinician transfigures into an elder statesman. Admired by many and despised by some the senior figure begins to occupy a larger space within the territory, and in some cases displays pomp and grandeur, or even dominance over other species or other members of his class. The following joke that I have heard as well as regurgitated a few times at surgeon-friendly get-togethers sets out the theme.

An internist, an ER physician, a surgeon, and a pathologist decided to take a break from the hospital and went duck hunting together. Next morning, they were sitting in a duck blind waiting for the birds. Eventually, one appeared on the horizon.

The internist watched it carefully, and as it came over in a leisurely manner he whispered, "Gentlemen, notice the colourful plumage, the distinctive quacking sound, and the web feet trailing behind."

As the bird flew out of range, raising the tone of his voice he added, "Based on my observations, I would venture that we have seen a duck, but we cannot be absolutely certain."

The other doctors looked at the internist, then at each other, and then turned their attention towards the sky again. It wasn't long before another bird appeared. They waited until it came closer. Excitedly the ER physician yelled, "It's a swan! No, it's a goose! No, no wait! It's a duck!" He whipped out his gun and fired multiple rounds into the air, each one missing the target. Alas, the bird flew away.

When the next bird flew by, without saying a word, the surgeon stood up took aim, and shot. The dead bird fell into the blind. And then he turned to the pathologist and said, "Old chap, could you run over there, get that damn thing and tell me if it was a duck?"

Joking apart, the fact is that a surgeon should possess the ability to act decisively in unexpected and time-limited situations, and have the talent to improvise if necessary. Furthermore, to make a cut and lay open a fellow human is in itself a testing undertaking, which requires a robust and resolute mind. All these attributes create the aura around a surgeon. The ambience is magnified further by the very nature of the job. Confirmation to a patient and the family that the operation was a success makes the person a champion in the eyes of those who hear that pleasing news. The clinician becomes the subject of conversation amongst friends, family and colleagues – during dinner parties, club meetings, afternoon teas, pub get-togethers, etc. Praises are showered with phrases like: very good chap – top class in his field – thorough in whatever he does – best in the business, and so on. Moreover, surgery is a result-orientated vocation that involves hands on skills, ranging from coarse manual tasks like hammering a nail into a long bone to delicate art as in microscopic and reconstructive surgery. In both cases the quality of work as well as the end result are on display – in front of trainees, nurses, theatre-personnel and of course patients and their loved ones. As a consequence showmanship blends into a surgeon's behaviour, which can reflect in many ways – body language, attire, walking style, mannerism, and speech.

While most surgeons exhibit showmanship of a varying degree, some are real show-offs. A few find pleasure in driving around in fancy cars and some try to make themselves noticeable by acquiring personalised number plates, usually linked to their field of practice. The results of a survey by elephant.co.uk revealed that surgeons topped the list of occupations owning personalised number plates, with a figure of over nine per cent. The plates that I have seen and heard about over the years include: TUR (transurethral resection) 11 *[urology]*, GYN H *[gynaecology]*, H4 TUM *[gastroenterology]*, ENT 1B & ORL 1 *[oto-rhino-laryngeology]*, P13 EYE & SEE 5 *[ophthalmology]*, THR (total hip replacement) 1, TKR (total knee replacement) 12 & HIP LR *[Orthopaedics]*, BOO8 *[cosmetic surgery]*, and BRA 1N *[neurosurgery]*.

There are also other ways to show off – some cannot resist worldly temptations and derive pleasure by wandering into the territories of others. An incident from my medical student days comes to mind.

Prof K was a general surgeon to the core – a larger than life personality with the expertise to tackle anything surgical. He was tall and muscular with a large body frame – much like a rugby prop. Moreover, he carried an air of authority around him and was respected and revered by his peers, pupils and patients. Abdominal surgery was his home ground and watching him perform an open prostatectomy was a treat. He could easily lift depressed fractures of skull, perform open reduction of fractures and undertake bone grafting. Sometimes he even dabbled into gynaecology.

On this day Prof K was operating in one of the theatres of a two-theatre complex. After having finished the operation in his theatre, like a lion patrolling the open plain, lazily he started strolling up and down the theatre-corridor. A newly appointed assistant professor working on a different firm was performing an emergency appendicectomy in the other theatre next door. He had opened the abdomen through the standard incision normally used for this procedure but was unable to locate the vermiform appendix and had already spent a long time on the case. The scent of blood made Prof K wander into the next-door theatre. On seeing the lord of the jungle the young surgeon became more unsettled and his task became even harder.

After watching the young man struggle for about five minutes Prof K could not resist the temptation. Without saying anything he put on a pair of sterile gloves, asked the operating surgeon politely to move to one side, picked up a surgical knife from the trolley and made another cut on the patient's abdomen at right angles to the original one. The incision now looked like the letter T. And *voilà!* – The appendix immediately popped out. There was a wow all round and at that point he moved away from the table gracefully with the comment, "Please carry on."

Appearing visibly embarrassed but thoroughly impressed, the assistant professor mumbled sheepishly, "Sir, I have neither seen nor read about this incision… Who described this T incision, sir?"

Without turning his head and with a contented smile on his large face the big boss replied, "Prof K, who else?" And he walked out and disappeared into the surgeon's room to have his favourite Gold Flake cigarette.

Every surgeon aims to achieve the position of eminence – to be the head of the pack and become the chief. Most chiefs reflect warmth and veneration from that position, but a few carry a steep authority gradient and emanate fear and unease. Many years ago I made a planned visit to a surgical centre of repute to learn about a procedure related to my specialty. I arrived in town the night before and received instructions from the second-in-command of the department to be in the conference room at 7am next morning. Arriving ten minutes early I was surprised to find that the room was already full, and everyone was seated in chairs around a very large table. Only the boss's chair was empty. It appeared like a politburo with everyone having a fixed spot around the table. The only place I could find for myself was alongside a couple of medical students who were seated on armless chairs at a fair distance outside the ring.

The room was unusually quiet and everyone was waiting expectantly for the big professor to grace the occasion. He was apparently an expert wildlife hunter and had been away – not on a hunting expedition but lecturing in some part of the world. Apparently he did that for more than half of the year. At a quarter past seven, a hush enveloped the room as an older looking man of average height with a deeply wrinkled face and a large head covered by a grey and thin tuft of hair, dressed in a bold pinstriped designer suit with a colourful bow tie, walked into the room.

Without any pleasantries he was straight on to business. He looked at his first assistant who was seated on his immediate right. Instantly the latter started the proceedings by saying a few softly spoken words, after which the boss began his address in a loud and gruff tone. Even though I didn't understand the language that was being spoken it was clear that by turns he was bombarding each person seated around the table. A lot of finger pointing was going on – there were no smiles and no jokes – everyone seemed alert and nervous. The meeting closed as abruptly as it had begun. Later in the day he showed up again, this time in the operating theatres. He went round each of the three theatres, and without saying much wrote a little note on each patient's notes and whizzed away.

Within a couple of days it became clear to me that the man behind the success and the aura for which this man was well known all over the world was actually Dr G – his second-in-command, who was a very competent surgeon. After a few days I became quite friendly with him and during the course of our conversation I said to him, "Do you know you possess a brilliant pair of hands; why don't you work independently without having to take the crap from the headmaster?"

In broken English with overstressed vowels Dr G replied with a one-liner, "My friend, he is the queen ant and I am the worker."

On hearing that I didn't think it proper to extend the conversation on the subject.

A small minority of surgeons from the masculine gender in

particular consider themselves to be alpha animals and the trait becomes particularly noticeable in their home ground – the operating theatres. Much like in the animal world, they expect to receive preferential treatment when they make themselves visible to other creatures. The situation becomes dire if two tigers wander into the same territory at the same time and start eyeing each other. The conflict can generally be resolved by crafty nurse managers, or friendly anaesthetists, or tactful juniors – or sometimes by all three. Occasionally the clash becomes a showdown that can end with one of the two licking his wounds.

TERRITORIAL DISPUTE (FROM SD, CARIBBEAN, 2003)

This was a Sunday morning and I was the anaesthetic consultant on call at one of the teaching hospitals in the West Indies. One of the obstetricians phoned the theatre sister regarding a lady who was in labour and needed emergency caesarean section (CS). However, a few minutes before that the surgical team on call had already booked the theatre for a patient needing emergency appendicectomy. Since CS is more urgent than appendicectomy I decided to allow the obstetrician to do his case first.

Both surgeons arrived in theatre at the same time and when the general surgeon learnt that he had been demoted to second position, he became berserk and demanded that his case was done first. A robust argument followed between the two surgeons. The general surgeon was saying that he had booked his case first and therefore he should have the first bite of the cherry. "I will not let you jump the queue, and mind you I will be in and out of theatre in half an hour." He was arguing vehemently.

The obstetrician was unwilling to budge and was saying repeatedly. "A caesarean is much more urgent than appendicectomy, you know that, don't you?"

Like parents unable to control two kids fighting over a toy, theatre sister and I watched the tussle while standing helplessly in theatre corridor. After a few minutes whilst the squabble was still going on, I moved away from the scene discreetly and asked the porters to wheel in the lady scheduled for CS. On seeing the patient being wheeled in, the general surgeon became more upset and dashed into one of the operating rooms, lay down on the operating table and declared, "I am not leaving this table until my patient is brought into this theatre."

We all left him there and whilst he continued with his protest by occupying one of the operating tables, theatre sister and I opened the second theatre where the obstetrician performed the CS. After a little while the general surgeon realised what had happened and disappeared from the scene quietly and returned an hour later, when his case was sent for. Unsurprisingly, there was pin-drop silence in the operating room during the appendicectomy. The surgeon did not speak to me for several months after the incident.

Although used sparingly nowadays, the use of the word God as a substitute for a male surgical chief was not uncommon in the days gone by. "We better get everything in order folks; God is returning from his hols and will be doing a ward round at 8am in the morning," the sergeant major (senior registrar or chief resident) would announce to the team.

I have often wondered why and how the word God got tagged onto surgeons. Moreover I have never heard the word Goddess being used for a female surgeon. I decided to look it up on the Internet, which was unhelpful but the exercise unearthed a few jokes and satires about the subject. One went like this.

After their death by some strange miracle, two lawyers made it to the screening area to procure permits for entry into the heaven. Whilst Saint Peter was checking their papers, he said to them, "Well, gentlemen, to enter the pearly gates you will have to stand in a line, and your position will be determined by how much you contributed to humanity during your lifetime. Let's face it, you're lawyers; you will have to wait patiently at the end of the line."

After talking to each other the lawyers agreed to stand at the end of a long and slow moving queue. They decided not to complain since they were able to look down into hell through the clouds and were able to watch from a distance how their partners were being treated there.

After a while, along came a surgeon in his scrubs wrapped in a flowing, majestic, open white coat. Carrying a bag and a mug of coffee, he walked right past the confused lawyers, along the line and up to Saint Peter. He nodded at the Saint, who nodded back, and walked through the pearly gates and right into the heaven – without being stopped or questioned along the way by anyone.

The lawyers, disgruntled at the fact that a surgeon had gone in before them, went up to Saint Peter and asked, "Your Holiness, what is special about that surgeon who bypassed everyone and went in without waiting in a line?"

Saint Peter replied, "Oh, Him? That was God himself. He likes to think he is a surgeon sometimes."

Back on earth how does the society perceive surgeons? In Asia during surgical consultations it is quite common for patients as well as their loved ones to make statements like: 'After the Almighty, I am in your hands,' 'Everyone says that God has blessed you with *dast-i-shifa* (healing hands),' 'You gave me a new lease of life; for me you are like God,' and so on. The famous BBC TV documentary series that examined surgical practice from the point of view of surgeons as well as patients, was entitled *Your Life in Their Hands*. It follows that in all cultures a surgeon is perceived to be a facilitator of the Godly act of saving a life. That may be so but that is certainly not the reason for esteeming a surgeon with the divine title. Do surgeons behave in an omniscient manner and treat others as mere mortals and do they develop a sense of detachment as they grow in stature?

The reality is that for the vast majority it is a privilege to be a surgeon, get involved in someone else's life and be able to make a difference. Barring rare exceptions, the surgeons that I rubbed shoulders with in my life, were highly skilled, hardworking, dedicated, compassionate and caring professionals. It is also true that the aura around a surgeon sprouts naturally out of real respect and even adoration for the ability and qualities of the individual, and the end result of actions displayed by the person repeatedly in testing situations over a period of time.

In 2011 the Canadian Urological Association conducted a study on personality traits of surgeons versus non-surgeons, and urologists versus other surgeons. It concluded that all surgeons (surgeons as well as urologists) were more extroverted than non-surgeons but the urologists were more extroverted than other types of surgeons. Interestingly no significant differences were observed amongst the three groups with regard to openness, conscientiousness, agreeableness and neuroticism. It is probably the extroverted and assertive aspect of a surgeon's personality that is overplayed and probably misperceived. It is, however, important to point out that a fine line separates assertiveness from arrogance. Not only is arrogance a bad character trait but also dangerous when it comes to surgery. A combination of arrogance with incompetence forms a toxic cocktail that is a recipe for disaster in a surgical setting.

It is said that surgeons have a stereotypical surgical personality. What does the term mean? Is it the one that is currently depicted on various television channels in serials like *Casualty*, *ER* and *Holby City*, of a well-groomed, well-spoken, hardworking, compassionate, dashing and handsome individual (usually a man!)? Or is it the character invented more than half a century ago by the film gurus of that period who showed a surgeon as a brash grandee – demanding, dominating and daunting, with a bulky frame and a bellowing voice – the role played admirably on the screen by James Robertson Justice in the popular series of *Doctor* films? Having watched both the old and current series it is clear that in both eras a surgeon has been portrayed as a team leader. However, the public image of a surgeon depicted on the screen during the 1960s and 70s was completely different to the one in the twenty-first century. The reality on the ground was no different either; in the bygone era the world was inhabited by a small number of surgical personalities who suffered from God-complex syndrome that manifested itself in different forms in the clinical arena.

GOD'S WORD IS LAW (FROM JV, UK, 1981)

This was my first junior surgical posting and I had been in post for about 2 months. One morning during his routine weekly ward round the boss (Mr G) noticed that out of the total of twenty patients on the male ward five had laboratory documented urinary tract infection caused by the same species of bacteria. After seeing the last patient on his ward round Mr G summoned the hospital administrator to the ward and said, "There is too much infection on this ward; therefore I have decided to shut the ward from now on." And with that sentence he along with his entourage (which included me) walked off to see rest of the patients who were scattered in other parts of the hospital.

By mid-morning we finished the ward round and returned to his office, which was close to the 'infected' ward. By then the administrator, senior microbiologist, head of facilities and surgical nursing officer had arrived on the scene and were huddled together in the centre of the ward working out a plan of action. Little did they know what was coming next!

After having his post-ward-round cup of tea and biscuits Mr G summoned the administrator again and announced: "We need to take off all doors and handles from toilets. These old boys open the toilet doors with their hands and that is how they transmit infection to one another."

The order was followed without questions; in came the carpenters who removed doors and door handles from the toilet doors. Patients were distributed to other wards in the hospital; deep cleaning was started under the close scrutiny of the microbiologist. All routine admissions were cancelled. The situation eventually returned back to normal after two weeks.

Imagine this happening today; there would be an emergency meeting involving all stakeholders – the secretaries would have a hard time rescheduling diaries. A brigade of managers would arrive for the meeting with their notebooks and laptops. Arguments would flow to and fro and after the debate the likely decision would be to review the situation in a week or more – and by then the issue would be forgotten.

Gods do not err (from BI, UK, 1975)

Cramming together of multiple gallstones within the gall bladder tends to flatten some of their surfaces. Occasionally some stones spill over into the common bile duct (CBD) – the tube that drains fluid from the gall bladder and liver into the bowel. That necessitates surgical exploration of the duct at the time of gall bladder removal (cholecystectomy).

Before the era of keyhole surgery, exploration of the CBD was undertaken frequently and the surgeon would place a T shaped rubber/latex tube, with the short arm of the tube inside the duct and the long arm connected to a bag or a bottle outside to drain bile. The T Tube would be removed after a few days, but before removal radiopaque contrast liquid would be injected into the tube to be absolutely certain that there were no stones left in the CBD during the initial operation.

I worked as a junior for a London surgeon who prided himself on his infallible surgical technique. He was quite annoyed to find that following the above procedure the radiologist had reported that the post-operative X-ray showed three residual stones in the CBD.

Gods do not err, and they do not leave stones behind, and therefore he, along with the team of his disciples – that included me, marched to the radiology department and pointed out to the radiologist that the defects on the X-ray were not stones but air bubbles that might have been introduced during injection of the dye. Even though everyone present except the boss thought that the shadows were leftover stones, no one dared to contradict. How could they? That was God's word!

The humble radiologist heard the surgeon patiently and responded by saying, "I am awfully sorry; if you think this is an error I will issue a new report." Triumphantly the boss walked out of the radiologist's office and we all followed behind.

The written report from the radiologist arrived the following day and read as follows:

'There are three FACETTED BUBBLES within the common bile duct, differential diagnosis? – Stones, PS: Air bubbles are usually round, stones are usually facetted!"

GODS DO NOT LIE – THEY CAN BEND THE TRUTH
(FROM FK, UK, 1970S)

Mr T was a real personality – a brilliant clinician and surgeon who was loved by his patients and adored by the staff. He was in his early sixties. Being an ex-sportsman he had a strong physique and looked much younger than his age. His influence and reputation went far beyond the boundaries of the hospital where he worked. Whatever he said was accepted without any reservation by everyone.

I was a medical student attached to his unit for my clinical posting. A lady was being operated for open pyeloplasty – an operation to relieve the blockage in the upper end of the tube that connects the kidney to bladder. Mr T asked the registrar to begin the operation and expose the kidney while he sat in the surgeon's room chatting with his consultant colleagues.

The registrar exposed the left kidney after making a long cut in the patient's left loin. However, to his dismay he could not find any obstruction in the tube and therefore he called the boss for help.

Mr T immediately asked for patient's X-rays, which were hurriedly taken out of a thick bundle from a large envelope. Everyone in theatre was stunned when he exploded with anger with a barrage of words directed at everyone present, "You fools, you have exposed the wrong kidney; turn her over and we will open the other side."

There was a shocked hush all round. Like a bunch of robots everyone went through the motions quietly. The wound on the left side was closed and a dressing applied and the patient was repositioned with the right side up. Mr K got scrubbed and performed the entire procedure – this time on the correct kidney, that took him no more than an hour. The patient left the operating theatre with two long cuts, one in each loin. Everyone was devastated at the blunder.

Next morning Mr T came to see the patient on his rounds and greeted the lady with a smile and a handshake. She was very well and was merrily eating her breakfast. He explained to her with the help of a diagram what was done on the obstructed kidney.

After he had finished the lady asked nervously, "Mr T, I noticed I have got two cuts, one on each side…"

With a reassuring smile he replied, "So you have. I should have mentioned that we looked at your other kidney at the same time."

"Did you find anything sir?"

"No, I am pleased to tell you that the other side is perfectly normal," he said authoritatively.

"Thank you so much, Mr T, I am so pleased to know that," replied the lady. And with that Mr T shook hands with her and the team went on to the next bed.

GODS PREFER SILENCE! (FROM GM, 1990S, AUSTRALIA)

The incident happened at the start of my surgical training. On this particular day the boss, who was a well-respected surgeon in the circuit, was going to undertake a hernia repair on a man in his forties. While the anaesthetist was putting the patient to sleep the boss went to the beverage dispenser in the theatre suite and got himself hot coffee in a disposable plastic cup. Before he got a chance to start drinking it, the anaesthetist called him to the anaesthetic room to check the side where the hernia was present. As he leaned over the anaesthetised patient with the cup in his hand a few drops of hot coffee spilled on the patient's umbilicus. Being already anaesthetised the patient did not feel any pain. The area was wiped dry and the hernia operation proceeded uneventfully thereafter.

Next day the boss arrived on his post-operative ward round. The patient was absolutely fine with no discomfort from hernia repair. However, he could not understand why his belly-button area was painful and wanted an explanation.

On hearing this, the boss went into a state of bewilderment, appearing totally mystified, looked around and made eye contact with every member of the team who were standing around the bed. After a protracted period of silence he said, "That is something we need to reflect upon; meanwhile we will put some clean dressing on the area." Everyone maintained the code of silence.

The patient returned for follow-up two weeks later. By then everything had healed including the raw area on the bellybutton. In fact he had already forgotten about it and there was no further discussion regarding the incident either.

The characters described in the above anecdotes were all good surgeons, well known for their technical skills, but they lived and practised in an era when professional regulation was conspicuous by its absence. Since then the surgical world has undergone a transformation. During the closing years of the twentieth century a number of serious surgical mishaps caught the attention of the public in the West. In the UK it began with the Bristol Heart Scandal and after the disgraceful revelations about Rodney Leadward – self-dubbed "the fastest gynaecologist in the south," the public image of a surgeon sank to its lowest point. As the pressure for change mounted, over a period of time newer concepts of safety in healthcare emerged that began with the introduction of clinical audit and governance in surgical practice and culminated in the development of methodologies and tools for quantitative assessment of quality in healthcare – in particular surgical care. Calls for accountability and appraisal of surgeons resulted in strengthening of powers of the regulatory and advisory bodies. All these changes transformed the profile of surgery as a specialty. The document entitled 'Surgical Leadership' issued by the Royal College of Surgeons of England in 2014 stipulates that good surgical leaders must act with integrity, be honest and open, decisive and consistent, accessible and open to challenge and feedback, self aware and mindful of impact on others, and must recognise their own response to stress. The GMC document 'Good Medical Practice' emphasises that: 'You must make sure that your conduct justifies your patients' trust in you and the public's trust in the profession.' The all-knowing and all-powerful figure immune to scrutiny was slowly driven into a state of extinction.

6

THE THEATRE

The Operating Theatre (OT) – or theatre – also known as the Operating Room (OR) or Operating Suites (OS), is the epicentre of surgical drama and action. Before the advent of modern surgical practice it used to be a large room with a raised table or chair at the centre, which was used for performing various procedures on patients. Around the periphery of the room were a number of rows of seats, from where apprentices and spectators watched the case in progress. Like butchers, surgeons wore street clothes with aprons to protect them from bloodstains. They operated barehanded with unsterile tools, needles and strands of silk thread. I have seen an operating theatre at a mission hospital in Kashmir that was built at the beginning of the twentieth century, where an open gutter connected to an outside drain ran across the length of the operating room. The gutter was apparently used to wash off blood, pus and other body fluids.

The present day operating theatre is a highly sophisticated and technologically advanced complex that permits integrated deployment of all surgical and non-surgical gadgets and tools needed by the surgeon, the anaesthetist and the rest of the operating team.

Much like a play on a stage, in the operating theatre art, skill and experience blend together, and years of training, learning and education are put on display. The pressure to perform well is on the surgeon. There is no second-take, you have to get it right the first time. For that one requires a state of mind, which is clear, focussed and imaginative, and which has the ability to receive and decipher the resonances emanating in the background. In the infamous incident at the Welsh Hospital in 2001, the alarms raised by a medical student – that a wrong kidney was being removed, were deliberately ignored by the operating surgeon. The end result was a surgical catastrophe.

My regular anaesthetist Dr V – undoubtedly one of the best in his field, and I, have been working together week after week for more than two decades. Much like a married couple, we have been through our triumphs and tribulations together. One episode that remains engraved in my memory is when he forbade me firmly from closing the abdomen of a lady after I had undertaken left nephro-ureterectomy (removal of kidney and the tube connecting it to the bladder) on her. "Can you have a look again in the abdomen; something isn't right," he warned me with an unusually worried look on his face.

"What does he want me to do? I have already checked the operated areas." I thought to myself. However, I didn't say anything; instead, with the help of my assistants I inspected these areas again, and everything appeared okay.

Without looking into my eye, whilst he was busily giving instructions to his assistant he repeated, "I am telling you, there is something amiss, I don't know what; I can't maintain her blood pressure!"

Frustratingly I replied, "Are you sure that there is nothing wrong at your end?"

He probably heard my question but pretended otherwise and chose not to reply. I could, however, sense a deep anxiety on his face while his mind and body appeared fully engaged with the predicament that we both were in. Without waiting for his response

I started inspecting the abdominal and pelvic cavities again. On this occasion however, I asked the team to raise the head end of the operating table. Immediately after that a steady drip of fresh blood started welling up and as I followed its source, well away from the operated site I found a large pool of blood and clot wedged between the left hemi-diaphragm and liver, that had collected from a continuous dribble originating from a small capsular breach in the spleen. The collected blood was evacuated and the bleeding controlled. The patient made an uneventful recovery. My colleague not only saved the day for all of us, but also saved a life.

The lady saw me regularly for a number of years thereafter. At each follow up visit she and I spent a few minutes reminiscing about the episode. Dr V's name was of course mentioned every time during our conversations.

Some of the expressions and behaviours exhibited by surgeons in theatre are the outcome of a flow of adrenaline within their systems. Over a period of time these get tagged on to their neurological network and grow into habits. Some performances are purely artificial put on by the lead actor to get the job done, whereas some are involuntary outbursts of elation or anxiety brought on by minor surgical successes or difficulties. With time the whole supporting cast – the anaesthetist, operating department assistants (ODAs), theatre nurses and junior medical staff get used to them. Emotional peaks and dips generate light-hearted comments that no one takes seriously. However, some utterances convey a serious message that alerts everyone present.

Whenever I found myself confronted by challenging situations such as – when dissecting near large blood vessels in the pelvis during major pelvic surgery, or while removing a large kidney tumour abutting the main blood vessels like the aorta and inferior vena cava – I would look towards Dr V and announce, "Folks, we are in tiger country." I do not know how the phrase got embedded into my system – perhaps after watching too many David Attenborough documentaries. However, these words worked wonders; everyone present in theatre – whether scrubbed or not, became even more tightly focused and vigilant than they already were, until the job was accomplished successfully. It brought me other rewards too – I was overwhelmed to receive a tapestry wall picture specially made for me by my theatre staff on my sixtieth birthday, showing a lead tiger with four smaller tigers following behind in a file, along with a greeting card which read, "Beware, we are in the tiger country." The picture hangs proudly in my study. On one occasion after I uttered the catchphrase a newly appointed senior house officer of Sri Lankan roots, who was a spectator in theatre and was unaware of the significance and the seriousness of the situation, chipped in with the comment: "That is where I come from sir – Sri Lanka – they call it the tiger country. Sir, have you been there?" All eyes focussed their radar at him but no one said anything.

It is interesting to watch the working dynamics in an operating theatre and observe how well the team members are fine-tuned to one another's language – the spoken and the unspoken, and how they are able to decipher and differentiate distress calls from uneasy mutterings and casual quips by the surgeon. I used to work as a junior for a boss who would whisper the words 'for my sins' every few minutes during the course of an operation. Another colleague of mine had the habit of saying repeatedly, "Where can it be? It has to be there." When in difficulty, one of my bosses would start sighing deeply, and to reinvigorate his spirits and those of his assistants declare, " Chaps, no guts no glory." Another chief would reject a knife blade by saying, "This won't cut even through a piece of s***." A colleague remembers a female surgeon, who would for some reason moan about the surgical scissors in particular. The scrub nurses replaced these on a regular basis during the course of an operation. When the going became difficult she would utter the words, "Where do you buy these blunt instruments from – Mauritius?" In the following anecdote narrated by a colleague the surgeon was lucky to escape unhurt after enunciating his favourite catchphrase.

I AM STILL STERILE! (FROM *PJ, UK, 1997*)

I worked as a senior house officer for Mr Z who was the senior-most surgeon in the department. He was pompous by nature, had an edgy temperament and would transform into an emotional eccentric within the theatre environment. He would get excited with small accomplishments like after successfully fishing out a stone, or after easy removal of a diseased body organ. Worst still, he would become hyper-excited if the procedure turned out to be more complex than expected. With the increase in difficulty there would be a palpable rise in tension within the operating theatre. He would trot around in a circle, thump the floor hard with his right foot and bellow out the words, "I have never seen such anatomy before!" This somehow acted as his release valve and calmed him down – he would walk back to the table and carry on. The ritual would be repeated at intervals until the situation eased at the business end of the proceedings. With each of his cursing outbursts about the imaginary unusual anatomy the theatre staff would quietly whisper to one another, "Heard that before!"

One day he was rather overzealous with his rhythmic ritual to the point of losing his balance. He slipped and landed heavily on his massive buttocks on the hard concrete floor. He appeared dazed but kept his sterile gloved hands in the air, and after recovering his posture and pride, got up and declared triumphantly at the top of his voice, "Thank goodness, I am still sterile!" Fortunately he did not suffer any serious injuries but he had to scrub again to finish the rest of the operation. Needless to add, the incident did not alter his behavioural routine in any way.

An efficient operating theatre is like a well-oiled chain that moves smoothly, and that saves time and improves outcomes. The direction of the instructional flow is normally from the surgeon to the assistant/scrub nurse, and from the scrub nurse to the circulation nurse. I have asked a number of theatre nurses the question, "What makes a good scrub nurse?" In most cases the reply was to the effect, "To be able to anticipate the surgeons' next move before they make it." That can only happen if there is a sense of discipline all round.

The vast majority of surgeons are even-tempered and reasonable, and have the capability to absorb the shakes and sparks of a surgical journey during a complicated procedure, and are able to maintain a sense of calm, at least on the outside. However, some exhibit flashes of impropriety when they get to work in theatre. Reminiscing about her days as a scrub nurse a senior theatre sister from the UK narrated to me her experience about a surgeon who was very precise in his operating habits – his command had to be carried out without any argument. Once in a while his obsession went too far – if a particular instrument of his choice was not available, he would remove his gloves and sterile gown in a flash and disappear from the scene with the remark, "When you get the instrument, call me, I am waiting in the surgeons' room."

A small minority become awkward and irate in the theatre environment and sometimes blow a gasket making a theatre day long and thankless for everyone involved. Generally such a situation develops if the surgical voyage hits difficulties; like when the tissues are stuck, or the blood ooze doesn't stop, or the stone is difficult to grasp, or the angle of approach to the target area is awkward. And if the scrub nurse hasn't got a particular instrument or a suture, or a vital tool of choice on the trolley, the individual demands urgent attention. Interestingly, even without that crucial instrument in most cases the restless mind still manages to improvise and move on, but the fuse has been lit – and when the cautery starts working intermittently or the sucker doesn't suck efficiently or its bottle gets clogged up, or theatre lights do not illuminate the desired field of action, or the assistant becomes a hindrance instead of help, a state of chaos and confusion ensues, resulting in everyone in theatre becoming edgy. That is where the senior theatre sister – who has worked in that theatre or with that surgeon for years, comes to everyone's rescue. She (uncommonly he) acts as a balm for the troubled mind. Seeing the familiar and friendly face the surgeon takes in a deep breath and explodes with relief, "Where have you been Sister J? It has been a real struggle so far."

The calm and collected saviour – the mother superior – responds back with authority, "Just take a break for a couple of minutes; let's look at the diathermy and the sucker."

The screaming child shuts up, obeys the directive and after a few minutes miraculously the surgical ship starts sailing away smoothly across the serene sea.

As a rule, cases never go smoothly for a habitually angry surgeon. Swab or instrument counts become muddled, a needle is suddenly missing and a state of high tension prevails. Everyone scrambles to find the needle and a call is made for an X-ray to be taken in theatre. The surgeon is livid about the delay and insists that the needle couldn't be inside the patient and starts shifting the blame onto everyone else and decries the hospital managers and policy makers. Fortunately, the needle is soon found and no X-ray is required. Eventually the surgical procedure is completed and the patient is woken up from the anaesthetic. As soon as the irate soul leaves the theatre premises everyone breathes a sigh of relief and there are smiles all round. Time to prepare the stage for the next act as another lead actor walks in with a broad smile – the show must go on.

Anger is a state of temporary madness that makes a surgeon behave in an irrational manner. In the olden days angry surgeons – the vast majority of whom were males, used to throw instruments. The following examples of instrument throwing from the bygone period, recounted by colleagues from three different continents demonstrate that it used to be a worldwide phenomenon.

IN THE FOOTSTEPS OF THE MASTER
(FROM CB, USA)

I started as a surgical resident at a US teaching hospital during the late nineteen nineties. The chief – who was nicknamed the Godfather, had the habit of throwing instruments on the floor at the slightest provocation. One of the responsibilities of the circulating nurses was to pick up the discarded items. They went through the ritual without any qualm accepting that as a routine in a day's work.

Much to everyone's relief the patriarch retired and his Fellow – a well-mannered guy, was appointed in his place. However, for some reason the new incumbent underwent a sudden personality change. He started using swear words in theatre and began following his mentor's footsteps by throwing instruments on the floor. Little did he realise that the world around had changed; he was disciplined by the Hospital President and ordered to go on a course on anger management. He did not misbehave thereafter!

IN THE EVENT OF FIRE BREAK THE GLASS!
(FROM RJ, INDIA, 1992)

This was the beginning of my anaesthetic career at a teaching hospital in South India. Dr Q, a male orthopaedic surgeon was a challenge to work with and would get upset about trivial matters. One could never be sure when he would blow hot – all present would be on their toes and would endeavour to avoid such a situation. This was the second time for me to be involved with his theatre list.

The incident started with Dr Q asking a newly appointed scrub nurse, who was helping him for the first time, for a periosteal elevator (an instrument used for scraping the bone surface).

"Which periosteal elevator, sir?" The scrub nurse asked politely.

"I said, give me a periosteal elevator." He responded angrily without even looking at the nurse. However, the nurse repeated, "Which periosteal elevator, sir?"

"Nurse, periosteal elevator is a periosteal elevator. Don't you understand?" Dr Q yelled back.

"I have three different periosteal elevators on my trolley; which one would you like to use?" She replied assertively.

Like a match to a leaky gas pipe the reply infuriated Dr Q. He stopped what he was doing, covered the wound with a large swab, moved towards the nurse, broke a theatre window pane with one of the orthopaedic tools, lifted the tray packed with instruments, threw it out of the window and walked out of theatre without saying a single word. Everyone was stunned and I felt listless.

The theatre manager came in, glass pieces were gathered, the window was temporarily sealed, and the scrub nurse and instrument trollies were changed – all with military precision. Dr Q returned to the scene and the procedure was completed, as if nothing had happened.

At the end of the procedure my anaesthetic boss said to me, "You look terrified."

"Yes sir, I am, I don't know what to say," was my honest reply.

"That is nothing new for us. He has been working at this hospital since the sixties and during these years he has broken several panes – if you look carefully in this theatre you will see that some panes are of different colours and textures." After a pause and with a satisfied grin he added, "He is retiring at the end of the month. Thank goodness for that!"

"Thank goodness for that!" I muttered to myself.

INDIFFERENT AND INSENSITIVE (FROM FR, UK, *1988*)

I had just started as an SHO and was working for Mr G, who was performing a complicated open abdominal operation on a grossly overweight man in his late sixties. I was the second assistant for the procedure.

Things were not going well at all and everyone was trying to make the situation easier for the boss, who was normally a cool customer, but because of the difficulties encountered he was getting increasingly irritable and twitchy. He started telling off every one and was blaming his assistants and anyone that he could think of.

He asked the scrub nurse for a scalpel to incise the tissues that he had exposed. With the scalpel held between his right thumb and two fingers he moved his hand close to the tissue to be incised but just before making the cut he changed his mind. He withdrew his hand from the area suddenly and instead of handing the scalpel back to the nurse he threw it onto the instrument trolley. Sadly, it hit the scrub nurse's hand and made a cut in his finger. Slowly his gloved hand started filling with blood – he clearly needed attention. He removed the gloves, applied pressure with a swab to the injured area and walked off whilst another nurse started scrubbing for the case.

There was complete silence in theatre. Mr G remained unmoved for about five minutes but then his patience ran out. Without realising that another nurse was getting ready in the washing area he shouted, "Can I have another scrub nurse please?"

For a tiny minority the theatre environment alters the settings on their verbal communication controls and they start using swear words whilst operating, with varying degrees of severity. It must be said that swearing is not a worldwide phenomenon and is conspicuously rare in hospitals in the East. However, in western hospitals one does come across surgeons, invariably males, for whom the utterance of a swear word acts as an outlet to their in-built tensions, and like other things it then becomes a habit. For some swearing is a component of the *prima donna* culture incorporated into their personality make-up.

Words like *God* or *hell* are not uncommon. A colleague recalls her female boss engaging a forceps to a baby's head during a difficult vaginal delivery and as she exerted a sustained pull she screamed at the top of her voice, "*Bloody hell*, you are coming out."

Swear words can include terms involving bodily products like *s***/p**** or seriously rude and abusive words like *f**** and *b****rd*. A study published in The British Medical Journal in 1999, involving one hundred consecutive surgical operations from five surgical specialties, revealed that the habit is more common in some specialities than others, with orthopaedics leading the field.

I enquired from a number of my surgical friends and colleagues if they swear during operating. I asked those who answered in the affirmative why they resorted to this practice and got a number of interesting responses.

"I never swear when I am concentrating or if I have a difficult job in hand. I swear only when I am relaxed and am doing something very routine. I do it out of affection. Trust me they, I mean my theatre staff, don't mind it."

"Swearing is a tradition in theatre, I guess it has become a routine for me. You should have heard my old boss, he would swear like a sailor; I am nothing compared to him."

"I swear only when I am in deep *s****, or when my assistants in theatre are clumsy. Besides, I know and they know that I don't mean it."

"You know in theatre we are all mates, real mates, we finish the day and go for a pint together – we crack dirty jokes and go home happy; you can ask them, they don't mind my swearing at all."

"Come to think of it, I have never thought of it. I agree it is a bad habit to swear whilst operating – I guess it is like an addiction, easy to acquire but hard to beat."

The incidence of swearing appears to be more common in some hospitals suggesting that it is more of a cultural issue within that institution. A surgical registrar who worked at my institution and who was subsequently appointed to a consultant post at another hospital in the UK met me at a conference many years later. He was a decent fellow who would never use a swear word whilst he worked at our place, but when I met him I soon realised how much he had changed – he would swear incessantly and blurted a swear word every couple of sentences, which made me uneasy to the point of saying to him: "You never used to swear when you were with us."

He replied, "I think you are right, the trouble is that every surgeon at our place does that." I guess I have been contaminated." He added laughingly.

On another occasion I had to interrupt a recently appointed junior male consultant colleague for repetitive abusive swearing, "That is disgusting. Is that how you speak in front of your family and children at home?" I asked. The guy never swore again – at least not in front of me.

The habit of swearing was more common with male surgeons of the older generation. The increasing use of local and regional anaesthesia is enforcing restraint on the surgical tongue although surgeons sometimes forget that under such circumstances their patient can be wide awake. The General Medical Council document 'Good Medical Practice' stipulates doctors to be 'polite and considerate'. In 2013 a surgeon who lost his temper, shouted and swore at colleagues and threw pieces of equipment, was suspended from the UK Medical Register for 12 months.

With tightening of the regulatory framework in recent years, examples of uncivil behaviour outlined above are becoming rare in the UK. The truth is that present day operating theatres are lively places where art and fun blend into a happy amalgam of fulfilment for everyone – surgeons, anaesthetists, junior medical staff and rest of the theatre team.

The vast majority of days in theatre are enjoyable, and each theatre day is a happy pill for all. The team come to know one other quite well and a state of informality evolves over a period of time. There is tittle-tattle gossip and loose talk about friends, acquaintances, competitors and colleagues, about latest scandals, hearsay rumours and political headlines within the patch, exchanges about politics, holidays, investments, stock market gains losses and predictions, sports and sporting bets, and much more. Being the lead actor, the surgeon starts the conversation but only if there is a relaxed mood all round – in other words when things are going well. It is usually not at the beginning of an operation and never when the surgical terrain is tough and tortuous. Light-hearted comments are quite common, and these help to gel the team together. Jokes flourish, which can sometimes unwittingly border on vulgarity but that works well in the vast majority of cases. Gaffes, funny actions and amusing incidents – intentional or otherwise – keep the whole theatre team on their toes, and maintain smiles on their faces.

I remember a senior surgeon who was grossly overweight and had a large protuberant belly. He had to use an XXXL theatre uniform that was specially made for him. Despite tightening his pyjamas well above his belly button, during the course of a long operation these would slowly slip down and once the knot rolled over the most convex point on his tummy, the pyjamas would crash on to the floor. One of the theatre helpers who had worked there for years would craftily manoeuvre under the surgeon's sterile gown, move the pyjamas back up his lower limbs over the tummy hump and tie the knots again. The ritual was sometimes repeated several times during a longer procedure. The team members were conditioned to this and the only people who found it funny were medical students – of whom I was one. I wondered why he did not use elastic waistbands?

A colleague who is now a consultant surgeon in the UK described to me his first day on a new job as a junior in a new hospital. This was his first case as the first assistant with the new boss. After a few minutes of starting the case his pyjamas slipped down. Since he had the habit of removing his underpants when changing for theatre, his buttocks were exposed. The news spread and during their breaks staff from other theatres dropped in to get a glimpse of his rear. Notwithstanding that, he maintained his concentration and remained adamantly stuck to his job until the long procedure was finished. Was he not bothered? I asked.

"I was hugely embarrassed, but did not want the boss to be annoyed with me. You know that was my first day of work with him."

A senior theatre sister described to me a bizarre incident of a large Mayo needle (a curved needle used for stitching tissues together) slipping out of a surgeon's needle holder, shooting up and almost reaching the theatre ceiling. The surgeon, who was a good cricketer in his younger days, dived towards his left with an outstretched hand and caught the needle. After acknowledging applause from the onlookers and shouts of "good catch" he fixed the needle back into the holder and carried on with the rest of the operation. In a similar incident recounted by a Spanish colleague a piece of bone graft taken from the ileum (hip girdle) that was to be grafted into the shoulder with a screw, flew off from the surgeon's hand into the air. The narrator, who was the first assistant, dived and caught the piece before it fell to the ground.

Some episodes or gaffes are particularly funny and are remembered for a long time after the event.

BLOOD AND SWEAT (FROM CF, UK, 1995)

It was a hot summer's day. The operation list had gone like clockwork – seven cases with no hiccups or complications. The last patient on the theatre table was a rather unfit gentleman who was undergoing transurethral resection of prostate (TURP).

It was not unusual for the department to have visitors from abroad, who were designated as clinical observers. On this occasion a Frenchman was attached to the unit for a two-week assignment.

A few minutes after the start of the operation the patient started bleeding from the prostate and as the procedure progressed the bleeding became worse. With increasing blood loss the operation was becoming progressively difficult and with that the surgeon's irritability index started going up, which was exhibited by large beads of perspiration on his forehead. Warm weather did not help. Everyone was quiet in theatre and the whole atmosphere was rather tense, when out of the blue the Frenchman said to the boss in a very polite tone, "Sir, could I wipe the sweat from your foreskin?" There was a roar of laughter, which broke the silence and relaxed everyone present.

The boss, who was known for his good sense of humour, replied, "Not now old boy, do it later."

Without realising the gaffe, the French doctor replied, "Okay sir, no problem."

ACTUALLY – IT WAS ME! (FROM WJ, POLAND, *1999*)

I was anaesthetising a fifty years old lady with the provisional diagnosis of intestinal obstruction secondary to bowel adhesions following previous abdominal surgery. The lead surgeon was one of the assistant professors but the chief of the surgical unit was also in attendance in the operating theatre. Expectedly the bowel was distended and as the adhesions were being separated and bowel moved from one side to another, there was a short whistling noise (like a fart) suggesting an air leak from somewhere in the bowel.

"I heard a noise, I think there is a small perforation in the bowel which you need to locate and close," advised the professor, after which he departed.

With that command the search for the hole in the bowel began in the earnest, but after inspecting the bowel loop by loop for about half an hour the leak could not be located. Wearily the operating surgeon said, "Can we call the professor please?"

At this point the scrub nurse interjected, "Please do not call him. Actually it was me, who made that noise. Sorry, I couldn't control it."

THE HANDICAP (FROM GH, SCOTLAND, 1971)

The story happened when I was a final year medical student. In those days, as part of the obstetrics learning, medical students had to carry out a set number of deliveries. A fellow student and I were assigned to a neighbouring hospital for our obstetric experience. The catchment area of that hospital was not the most salubrious in those days.

My colleague was delivering a young lady under the watchful guidance of the boss and the midwife. He was naturally nervous, and was so relieved to have successfully undertaken his first delivery that he said to the mother the first thing that came into his head, "Your baby does not have any hair, does he take after his father?"

In a deep Scottish accent the mother replied, "I do not know love, he never took his cap off."

Everyone present chuckled, the student didn't know what to say, but everyone learnt not to make comments about appearances with patients.

PART OF THE FAMILY (FROM TP, INDIA, 1994)

I was working as a surgical resident those days. There was an uprising going on and a protest march ended up with a pitched battle between the army and protestors. We were working in four operating theatres whilst the injured were being brought in. We had started in the morning and finished at 2am next day. Everyone including the chief, the middle faculty, surgical and anaesthetic residents, the anaesthetist (Dr K) and theatre staff had worked non-stop for almost sixteen hours. All of us were tired and exhausted.

Still in our theatre greens we assembled in theatre waiting bay when suddenly the boss undid his theatre shirt and pyjamas and stood completely naked. Everyone was smiling but no one dared to say anything to him. He went on talking about various patients and their clinical management, when hesitantly one of the assistant professors ventured to speak in a muffled tone. Pointing towards Dr K – who was the only female amongst us, he said, "By the way sir, Dr K is also standing here,"

'So?" he replied.

"You are showing, sir."

"What do you mean I am showing, what am I showing," he said loudly.

"You are showing, sir," repeated the assistant professor.

And then the penny dropped. He became uneasy and tried to cover his grey hairy privates with his hands but responded wittingly, "Oh! You mean... Dr K, ... she is one of us, she does not mind seeing me naked – I mean she is one of our own."

Dr K blushed and left the scene in disgust without saying anything.

The most memorable gaffe that happened in my operating theatre was when I was operating on a seventy-year old gentleman for transurethral resection of prostate. He had been put to sleep by the anaesthetist, positioned on the operating table and draped with sterile towels. The first stage in the procedure involves inspection of the inside of the bladder with an endoscope that is negotiated through the urethra (water passage).

As I started introducing the endoscope into the urethra, I noticed the patient developing a penile erection. Despite that I did manage to inspect his bladder, albeit with some difficulty. Following that I started negotiating a resectoscope – the instrument used to ream away the prostate and remove the prostatic bits per urethra, without the need to make an open cut. However, I could not negotiate it into the bladder, because by then the patient had developed a full-blown erection. The more I tried the more difficult it became, as the urethra became longer and the instrument appeared to become shorter. Frustrated with my inability to navigate I started looking for help but before I said anything my anaesthetist – the good old Dr V asked me, "What is the problem?"

"My problem is erection – can you help in anyway?" I replied after a pause.

By the time I muttered the above response to his question he was already seated on his stool at the head end of the table and was busily absorbed with his paperwork and chose to ignore me.

The rather diminutive scrub nurse was standing behind the patient's bent left leg and was busily arranging her instrument trolley. Completely unaware of the state of affairs at the business end of the operating table, her auditory sensors registered my plea for help. She moved closer to the table and asked me rather innocently, in a soft whisper, "Do you have a problem with erection, Mr M?"

"Just look at what is going on down there!" I said to her with a sarcastic laugh.

"Oops! Didn't realise, I thought it...it... it was you, I am extremely sorry," she tried to explain.

Mercifully the patient's erection abated and the procedure was completed without any problems, but the catchphrase – 'I thought it was you' – was repeated many times over in that theatre for many months thereafter.

Regardless of the length or complexity of the task in hand, a surgical operation entails organisation and planning. As a general rule the steps of an elective operation are well known and follow a set route that the surgeon has travelled many times before. The theatre team also know the journey well and are well prepared. Even for emergency procedures they are generally clear about the direction of travel but sometimes a change of plan is necessary. How well the team copes with the unexpected, tests the ability, resilience and lateral thinking of the lead actor as well as the supporting cast. Sometimes skills other than surgical save the day.

A BRIGHT IDEA (FROM SS, IRAQ, 1996)

I was the registrar on call in obstetrics at the large maternity hospital in Baghdad. During the early hours of night I decided to take a patient to theatre for emergency Caesarean Section because of failure of progression of labour resulting in foetal distress. After opening the abdomen and incising the uterus I managed to deliver a healthy baby. However, soon after that there was a sudden power failure, something that was not uncommon at that time due to lack of resources and destruction of the infrastructure after the First Gulf War. The whole hospital including theatres was pitched into darkness. In such circumstances normally the generator light would come on but on this occasion that didn't happen. To make matters worse there was no torch in theatre and not even a candle on hand – but there was a box of matches in a staff member's pocket.

I asked two circulating staff members to stand – one on each side of the table – and burn pages from the case notes of the patient alternately, page after page. The light emitted by the paper flame was bright enough for me to deliver the placenta, close the uterus and the abdominal wall, before the supply of paper and matches ran out. The patient survived and, the mother and baby were discharged home without complications.

A DIFFICULT AMPUTATION (FROM GS, UK, 1993)

One of my colleagues was carrying out an emergency above-knee amputation for an ischaemic (bloodless) leg. On sawing through the femur (thigh bone) he encountered unexpected resistance. Unbeknown to him the patient had fractured his femur in the past and had a Kuntscher nail (a stainless steel rod) put down through the entire length of his femur. Attempts at pulling out the nail failed; the solid nail needed to be transacted to get the leg off. Orthopaedic operating theatre was contacted for help but they had nothing to offer that would cut through the steel nail.

The surgeon hastily dispatched his senior house officer – still dressed in his theatre clothes – to a B&Q store to buy a suitable hacksaw that would be able to stand the extreme heat involved in the sterilisation process. The store staff was bemused by her appearance. Fortunately the B&Q hacksaw was up to the job and after a delay of about two hours the dead leg was taken off after the nail was transacted.

FIRE FIGHTING (FROM RB, UK, 1997)

The incident happened at a hospital in northern England where I was working as a registrar. A man in his early thirties who worked in the building industry attended the A&E in the middle of night with his penis stuck tight inside the hole of a ring spanner. Apparently the young man inserted his semi-erect penis inside the ring and after becoming excited the fully erect penis could not be retrieved. He was in pain with the spanner stuck at the penile root, the blood supply to the penis was getting compromised and it had turned blue.

After administering pain-relieving drugs the patient was shifted to theatre and put to sleep by the anaesthetist. I attempted to manipulate the spanner and release the penis, albeit without success. So I sought help from the consultant on call. He tried aspiration of blood from the engorged penis repeatedly to reduce its size but that also failed to alleviate the problem. So, he called the hospital engineer who arrived in theatre with his toolbox and tried to cut the metal with a metal cutter, but couldn't.

There was frustration all round and at this point the boss asked the team for ideas and one of the nurses suggested that we sought opinion from the local fire brigade. So he rang the local fire station. Initially he found it difficult to explain the purpose of his phone call because the fireman on duty thought that it was some weirdo making a hoax phone call in the dead of night, and hung up each time he was contacted. However, the hospital switchboard operator found the phone number of a high-ranking officer in the fire brigade department and put the call through to him. Half an hour later a team of firemen arrived on the scene with their metal cutting equipment.

Nervously and carefully the surgical and fire fighting teams worked together to cut the metal ring making sure that the cutter did not traumatise the engorged penis. There was a loud cheer when the penis was finally released from the noose of the strangling object. Luckily the penis survived the ordeal. At his follow-up appointment a few weeks later the patient's only complaint was slight discomfort during erection.

Like two actors who perform the same act differently two surgeons differ in their technique, style, mannerism, persona and skills. The operation may be the same, the team may be same, and the operating theatre may be the same, but the whole scenario is different if the surgeon is different. You could have a serious and pensive individual on a Monday and a loud and vivacious one on a Tuesday, a stern fellow in the morning and a sweet-tempered female surgeon in the afternoon. An irritant to one surgeon can act as healing balm for another. Some like a constant dose of their popular music number in the background. They confess that makes them work better and faster. Some prefer listening to the running commentary or ball-by-ball descriptions of their favourite sport on the radio. Some – like me, are unable to function effectively with noises in the background, musical or otherwise.

To a surgeon the operating theatre is what the church is to a clergyman, sea is to a sailor, war front is to a solider and stage is to an actor. You may have your own place of worship to pray, but this is the place where in my view you see glimpses of God. Each day is like a soap opera that brings on a new scenario, a new challenge and a new experience. This is the place where danger and delight grow together on one stalk. Regardless of the length or complexity of the task in hand, a surgical operation entails organisation, planning and teamwork. A surgeon is as good as the team that work with him/her and a team is as good as the systems that support it.

A well-knit team and a well-oiled system transform the day into a pleasant experience for everyone involved. Besides a good lead actor, a good production needs a fine-tuned supporting cast and a competent back stage staff. It is amazing though how theatre staff and anaesthetists adjust to changing surgical moods and temperaments, which alter with variations in the surgical landscape and the personality make up of the conductor of the orchestra. These dedicated men and women try their best to facilitate each step of a surgical procedure, because for them there is a single purpose – the welfare of the patient on the operating table. They deserve all the credit for their patience, resilience and perseverance.

7

FEMALE SURGEONS

One only needs to look around in the operating theatre of a western hospital to realise that the majority of staff working there are females, and most of them are nurses or operation department practitioners (ODPs). In Asian hospitals however, the scenario is different – a large number of males work as nurses and theatre assistants. As far as surgeons are concerned, there is a preponderance of males all over the world and because of that most stories about surgeons and surgery revolve around the masculine members of human species. Call it the boys' club or macho-culture there is no doubt that surgery has a masculine image – a central male character surrounded by a team of females in supporting roles.

The probable explanation for that lies in the development of surgery as an occupation and the evolution from a barber to a surgeon over the centuries. In the days gone by a barber was almost always a male who had the nerve to hold a sharp knife close to human flesh and move it effortlessly without causing damage and also use sharp instruments for procedures such as puncturing abscesses. Moreover, surgery demanded long and unsocial hours and it was generally the female partner who invested time in the upbringing of the family while the male went out to work. But has the scenario changed in recent years and is male domination of surgery on the decline?

The Edinburgh Seven were the first women to be admitted to the Edinburgh University to study medicine in 1869. One year later, an angry mob gathered at the Surgeons' Hall to prevent them from sitting their anatomy exam. There were no female surgeons at the close of the nineteenth century. A female British army surgeon, who was small in stature with feminine features, had to disguise herself as a male and become known by the name of Dr James Barry. He (she) was actually born and raised as a girl and was named Margaret Ann Bulkley. Among his (her) accomplishments was the first Caesarean section in Africa by a British surgeon in which both the mother and child survived. The deception was discovered only after her death but she was officially buried as a man.

Eleanor Davies-Colley was the first woman to acquire the FRCS (England) by examination in 1911. In 1919 there were only four female Fellows of the Royal College of Surgeons of England. Since then there has been a year-on-year increase in the number of female surgeons and the change is clearly reflected in UK surgical practice. The number of females with FRCS (England) was 320 in 1990 and this increased to 1,184 in 2009. In 2011 women constituted 8.7 per cent of the total consultant surgeon work force, and in 2014, 29.5% of surgical trainees were women. The proportional representation is also reflected in the composition of various surgical bodies in the UK. The current ratio of male to female members at the Council of Royal College of Surgeons of England is 16:5. The corresponding ratio at The Royal College of Surgeons of Edinburgh is 11:6.

In the US, the Association of Women Surgeons (AWS) was established in 1981. Its mission is "to inspire, encourage, and enable women surgeons to realise their professional and personal goals". In the UK, WINS (Women in Surgery) was established in 2007. Its mission is similar: "to encourage, enable and inspire women to fulfil their surgical ambitions".

According to the Royal College of Surgeons of England women are now represented in all nine surgical specialities and at all levels within a surgical career structure. The most popular specialty is general surgery with 37 per cent. Paediatric surgery represents 22 per cent of the female workforce. Interestingly, 15 per cent of female surgeons choose trauma and orthopaedics.

In the specialty of gynaecology and obstetrics, which deals exclusively with female patients, the situation is slightly different. The male to female ratio of officers of the UK Royal College of Obstetricians & Gynaecologists (RCOG) is 4:2. The office bearers of the Federation of Obstetric and Gynaecological Societies of India (FOGSI) have a male majority of 8:5. However, it is interesting that most of the office bearers of Society of Obstetricians and Gynaecologists of Pakistan (SOGP) are females with a majority of 12:1. The message from the previous president of that Society is heart warming and says it all: "For me this is a personal crusade, for me it is a debt I owe to the countless women who I have had the privilege to share my life with. For me it is pay back time."

The predominance of female gynaecologists in South Asia is also reflected in the staff structure at two well known institutions in that part of the world: All India Institute of Medical Sciences (AIIMS), New Delhi, India and Aga Khan University (AKU) Hospital, Karachi, Pakistan. At both institutions the faculties in the Department of gynaecology & obstetrics are predominantly female, in contrast with the departments of general surgery where it is predominantly male. There are cultural reasons for that – South Asian women prefer to seek advice from doctors of the same sex for gynaecological and obstetric problems.

Are female surgeons different from their male counterparts and do they have to behave differently to adjust in a male dominated playing field? I put this question to a number of my colleagues. The general impression is that the majority of female surgeons are stricter and tougher than their male counterparts but here are some thought-provoking stories from the front line.

TOUGH NUT WITH A SOFT CENTRE (FROM LJ, INDIA, *1985*)

This is an observational story that changed my own outlook to life as a doctor. I was working as a surgical trainee in a public hospital. My boss was a lady who everyone dreaded and that included many male surgeons. Poverty was everywhere; most patients and their families could barely survive on their meagre earnings – let alone afford medical care. They all ended up in public hospitals, where they were cared for without charge.

One such patient developed Stevens-Johnson syndrome due to a severe reaction to an antibiotic. The syndrome is characterised by cell death, which causes the epidermis to separate from the dermis. He developed ulceration of the whole skin and ulcers in his mouth that made it impossible for him to eat the hospital food and the family was asked to bring soft food cooked at home. Easier said than done – they could not even feed themselves.

Despite these difficulties the patient was doing surprisingly well – he was recovering; and slowly but surely his weight and blood parameters were improving.

The paradox was explained one day when I came in early for the ward round and found my female boss feeding the patient soft food cooked by her at home. Apparently this had been happening for many days before I found it out. None of us could have imagined that our formidable professor of surgery would prepare and bring along the much-needed soft food for this poor villager early morning every day. He made a full recovery and went home a few days later.

HE IS IN SAFE HANDS! (FROM GR, UK, *1996*)

The incident happened more than fifteen years ago at a private hospital where I worked as a nurse. The surgeon, Mrs T, was in her early sixties, short statured but elegant looking, and was known for her surgical expertise. She was gifted with nimble hands that would work craftily through difficult surgical territories. She had a dry sense of humour and would rarely smile.

On a late Saturday morning while she was in the middle of a major laparotomy (exploration of abdomen) the theatre sister answered an urgent phone call from the Emergency Department of the local NHS hospital. Mrs T's husband had suffered a heart attack.

Without informing Mrs T the theatre sister rang a male surgical colleague, Mr S at home and asked him to come in urgently to relieve Mrs T. Following that she went inside the operating theatre and said to Mrs T, "Sorry to interrupt you Mrs T, there is some bad news, your husband is in the Emergency Department at the NHS hospital. It could be a heart attack. I have asked Mr S to come in and help; he is on his way."

Looking over her half moon glasses with a fixed face and a stern look, she replied angrily, "You should have asked me first, sister!"

Then she paused for about thirty seconds, lifted her head again and said, "Please phone back Mr S, thank him on my behalf and tell him not to bother." And after another pause she added, "I know my husband is in safe hands."

Mrs T carried on with the operation without even raising an eyebrow. It took her a couple of hours to complete the procedure after which calmly she wrote the operation notes, spoke at length with the patient's husband outlining what she had done, and then drove to the other hospital to see her husband.

THE SQUEAMISH MISS (FROM KK, INDIA, 1998)

I was working as a senior resident for the only female general surgeon at the teaching hospital. She was an able clinician, an accomplished operator and a strict disciplinarian and had joined the department recently after training abroad. All her male colleagues kept a distance from her and juniors were generally scared of her.

One day she was operating on a young girl for small bowel obstruction and I was her first assistant. After opening the abdomen she discovered that the cause of the problem was a ball of round worms obstructing the small bowel lumen. As she manipulated the lump the serpentine movement of worms within the gut made her shriek at the top of her voice. She left the operating table and almost passed out in the corridor. I had to complete the rest of the operation. She admitted later that she was petrified at the sight of creepy crawlies. From then on every patient walking into the clinic or her ward had to be dewormed before any elective surgery was scheduled.

A PLEASANT NIGHTMARE (FROM SC, PAKISTAN, 2004)

I used to work as a registrar for a female professor of surgery at a teaching hospital in my country. She was a pleasant nightmare – soft mannered, sharp but single-minded. I had to get used to her hits on my knuckles with instruments on a regular basis whilst assisting her. She would continue with that until I mastered an action exactly the way she wanted. If she discovered that an intravenous cannula with adhesive tape had been left on a patient longer than necessary, she would stick a piece of adhesive tape on the most hairy part of a junior's forearm and then take it off so that the junior appreciated how painful that was.

A young man with acute intestinal obstruction secondary to bowel obstruction had to be operated by her three times for various surgical indications within a space of two months. Despite becoming quite unwell in the immediate post-operative period after each operation he recovered well. A week or so after the third operative procedure when he was almost ready to be discharged, sadly one morning he was found dead in his bed.

The female professor was given the news as she arrived for her ward round. She was devastated; she sat down in the middle of the ward and cried like a small baby. All staff members – doctors and nurses followed suit. It took us some time to console her and she took a week off from work. Life in the department didn't return to normal for many weeks after the event.

Do female surgeons use bad language and swear words like some of their male colleagues? As a general rule in most cultures men are louder and use bad language or swear words more often than women because swearing and abusive language is not considered to be lady-like. For some reason society tends to make harsher moral judgments about women. Swearing by females is not very uncommon in the western world but strangely enough I have never witnessed a female surgeon losing her temper or using swearwords. However, I have heard from several medical friends about lady surgeons who used abusive language and sometimes swear words when the going got tough in the operating theatre. A colleague remembered a lady who was not only a good surgeon but also a charming person under normal circumstances. However, on rare occasions when the going got too difficult she would first start telling off her team using uncivil words. If things didn't improve, she covered the wound with a swab, would move to one corner of the operating room, have a seat on a stool and have a good cry, whilst she was still in sterile attire. One of the nurses would gently wipe her tears and clean her glasses, following which she would get up and resume action without any further problems. Another colleague reminisced about a female surgeon who had the habit of blaming others for everything. She had a particular idiosyncrasy for hospital managers and her way of criticising them was rather peculiar. Whenever an opportunity presented itself, she would say, "It's no point talking to these managers. They can't even organise a piss-up in a brewery."

A recent book entitled, "Pathways to Gender Equality –

The Role of Merit and Quotas" concludes that notwithstanding the progress, overall, women's inclusion and representation in leadership roles (like surgery) remains slow. The evidence however, suggests otherwise. With better opportunities like flexible training, and flexible working hours, and with changing organisational and regulatory framework, more and more women are coming into the surgical fold. The current President of the Royal College of Surgeons of England is a lady orthopaedic surgeon. She was appointed in 2014 and is the first female president to be elected to this office in the College's 215-year history. Her election is a source of encouragement for women aspiring to be surgeons of the future. It also signifies a huge culture shift in the world of surgery.

8

THE JOURNEY

In many parts of the world most people rely on state-funded healthcare and it is not always possible to be cared for by a surgeon of one's choice. If you need an elective (non-emergency) surgical procedure you come to the nearest hospital or healthcare provider and get treated by whichever surgeon has the shortest waiting time. By and large, most patients like to be treated at their local hospital or health centre for non-emergency surgical conditions, unless the services of an expert in a particular field are required for which travel to a specialist centre becomes necessary. In the UK, and in many parts of the globe, an elective surgical journey begins with referral to a surgeon who the primary care physician considers as the most appropriate person for the job. Reports from friends, family and colleagues and word on the street about the overall reputation are also taken into account. Research interests, publications, clinical audits and writings by the surgeon indicate the position of the individual within the relevant peer group and provide information regarding training and experience. Hospitals in the West also publish quality accounts, patient experience surveys and inspection reports by the regulators. These give an idea about how well a hospital is managed and how good and safe the quality of care is. Advertisements by surgeons, hospital and personal websites, blogs and social media are also becoming increasingly important in surgeon selection. That is particularly so in US and Europe but the trend is catching up at a rapid pace in the developing world.

A small number of patients choose to travel from one country to another for surgical advice. In the past, patient flow used to be exclusively from less developed countries to major medical centres in the West; usually for high-end medical services and to have procedures or investigations that were unavailable in the home country. In a large number of cases that is still true. However, some travellers like the monarchs and Emirs from wealthy states in the Middle East, the rich and the famous, and those in higher echelons of power in the developing world, consider it a privilege – and in some cases a status symbol – to have a surgical operation or even an investigation, however simple, at a hospital in the West. London used to be a favourite terminus for such patients but as long distance travel became faster and more affordable, the US is taking over as the preferred destination.

During my junior days, assisting the boss at a private hospital used to be the unwritten part of the job description for a surgical trainee working in the London circuit. Such patients spent large amounts of money and were generally more demanding and also liked attention to detail. A senior colleague of mine, who also worked as a trainee in London, had to lend a sympathetic ear to a patient's wife who had reasons for being unhappy.

SHOP AROUND (FROM *BI, UK, 1986*)

As a senior registrar I worked for an eminent surgeon with an international reputation. I used to assist him in operations on his private patients at various London hospitals. On one such occasion the patient was a government minister in a Middle Eastern country. His wife and a party of officials and relatives accompanied him. The group was accommodated in a block of rooms at the hospital and a hotel nearby.

Unfortunately the patient developed post-operative complications, which necessitated a second operative procedure. His wife was most unhappy and the day after the second procedure she sought an urgent meeting with the medical staff. Since the chief was lecturing in a different part of the country on that day, the request was relayed to me.

I met a tall but oversized lady in the hospital director's office. Through an interpreter she conveyed to me her displeasure in no uncertain terms. With his eyes wide open, the interpreter – who was also from the Middle East and looked more like a nightclub bouncer, pronounced, "Doctor, you people need to know that Madam is most angry that her husband has to stay for longer than expected."

"Can you please say to Madam that one can never guarantee that an operation would go without complications, and can you also say that her husband is going to be fine?" I tried to explain.

"Madam says, that may be so but wishes to point out that they were actually planning to go to Paris for the operation, but it was she who had insisted to her husband that they came to London, simply because the shopping is much better over here. They have done all the shopping, but here they are, stuck for one more week – or who knows, may be for more than a week, with no more shopping to do."

I carried on giving assurances. Following the meeting I did not feel it necessary to pass on the details of the conversation to the chief.

The flow of international surgical tourism has, however, reversed in recent years with patients travelling from countries like the US, UK and the rest of Europe to developing countries in Asia. Notwithstanding the fact that clinical governance processes are non-existent and healthcare is largely unregulated in some of the countries, the business has been growing at a rapid pace during the last decade, mainly because of lower treatment-costs there.

Having chosen a surgeon and the hospital for a non-emergency procedure, the surgical journey begins. That can be a single or a series of encounters between the surgeon and the patient, and his family. In some cases the association can last a lifetime. For both the surgeon and the patient, however, a surgical operation is an experience – albeit of different kinds.

For the surgeon, in most cases the direction of travel is along a well-charted and frequently covered route. The exercise may be repetitive, but the terrain and road conditions vary, which offers the surgeon something new and different each time, thereby adding more miles to the individual's experience and expertise. The longer and more complex the procedure, the longer and more difficult is the travel, and therefore more important is the planning beforehand.

For the majority of patients it's a maiden journey clouded in nervousness or even uncertainty. Even when the outcome is expected to be favourable there are apprehensions about a number of issues such as: surgical failure, loss of personal control, pain during and after the operation, inability to wake up after the general anaesthetic and so on. It is also the fear of the unknown that overwhelms the anxious mind.

As a patient I had an encounter with a surgeon more than forty years ago. Soon after I tied my knot with the world of surgery a bout of lumbar pain unearthed an unpleasant surprise for me and my family – a 3cm stone was sitting in the pelvis of my right kidney, which needed to be removed surgically by a major operation. After getting over the initial shock, I looked for Mr S – the best cutter in town, who was known for his slickness and technique.

And there I was, sitting fretfully in his private consulting room with my dad seated by my side. My brain was working overtime thinking about the most rare complications that I might develop during or after surgery. What if there was excessive blood loss, or if I didn't wake up after the anaesthetic? I wasn't scared of the operation or of dying during the operation, but my main concern was pain. So, I plucked up the courage to ask the question, "Sir, will it be painful and how long will the incision be?"

Mr S replied with confidence, "Why do you worry about the incision? Good exposure needs a bigger incision, but we will make sure that you are not in pain." After a careful pause he added, "I wish there was a way to make a small hole to pluck out the stone, but I am afraid there isn't." The consultation was very reassuring and worked like a tonic that boosted my morale. I instantly went into a positive mode and wanted the stone out of my system as soon as possible.

The surgical procedure went well apart from a couple of small hiccups. When my surgeon was putting in the last two stitches to skin, the anaesthetist had probably already weaned me off the anaesthetic. I must have been in a state of trance – neither asleep nor awake, when I felt a needle going through my right loin twice in quick succession. That felt like two arrows piercing my body. The pain was excruciating – the worst I have felt in my life. Another instalment of pain was to follow a few days later, when a junior trainee removed the wide-bore rubber tube that had been left to drain any seepage from the kidney.

My surgeon wasn't aware about any of these events – on the first occasion I couldn't speak or move and on the second he wasn't there. I didn't bring it to his attention either. How could I? The authority gradient between him and me was too steep. Moreover, considering that the rest of the care was fantastic and I bounced back to full activity after three weeks, I thought it would be unkind and unwise to bring up these issues during the follow-up consultations.

More than thirty years later a young child of six, on whom I had undertaken circumcision, walked proudly into my follow-up clinic with his parents with a thank you card and a box of chocolates. The wording inside the card read, "Thank you for fixing me up great [sic]. All though [sic] it really hurt, all mum and dad went on and on about all the time how neat the stitching was."

They were all thankful but the youngster was telling me, in no uncertain terms, that he had been in pain. In a flash the child in me came to the surface as my thoughts slipped back to my painful moments when the scab and dry dressing came off my raw circumcision wound, and when I felt the sharp needle going through my freshly incised skin. I knew exactly what the child was telling me and I felt uncomfortable but without revealing what was crowding my neuronal pathways I asked him, "…Was it really painful?"

After looking at his parents, as if he was seeking their approval, he replied, "Yes, but I am okay now." He didn't change his mind – he had no reason to do that, but he was trying to be nice to me.

In contrast to the elective setting, in the case of an emergency the scenario is different. There is no time to lose and therefore there is no option except to seek advice from whoever is on duty at the nearest healthcare facility, regardless of the adequacy of the services available at that centre. In many cases the clinician and the team have no choice either; they have to deal with the emergency within the framework of the existing facilities and the experience of the team and the team leader.

After completing three years of surgical residency, I spent a few months at a quiet, suburban thirty-bed cottage hospital in Kashmir. Just after dusk on a Sunday evening, a young lady in her late twenties was rushed in as an emergency. She and her husband hailed from a big city in India hundreds of miles away. They were on their honeymoon in Kashmir. She had long and dense scalp hair intertwined into a single helix the lower end of which touched her lower back. The couple were enjoying a local lake trip in a primitive motorboat when suddenly her hair helix got entangled inside the blades of the wheel that turned the engine of the motorboat. Due to rotation at high speed her entire scalp was forcefully lifted and avulsed from her head.

It was a frightening scene. A few locals were carrying her; the helpless husband, who was smeared all over in blood, was carrying in his hands his wife's mud and blood soaked scalp covered with thick black hair. She was pale; her radial pulse was hardly perceptible and blood pressure was quite low. She had lost a lot of blood and blood was still pouring from the scalp edge all round her temples, forehead and occiput. The skull bone was completely bare.

I had neither seen nor read about total scalp avulsion before and didn't know what to do with the detached scalp but I realised that my immediate task was to save her life. So, I took her straight to the operating theatre and sent for the anaesthetist who lived nearby. At that hospital, arranging a blood transfusion during daytime on a weekday was a nightmare; on a Sunday evening that was impossible. Whilst my assistant and I put firm pressure on the wound edges all round the scalp, the anaesthetist who arrived on the scene straightaway, set up an intravenous drip and pumped fluids into her. As soon as her general condition improved slightly she was put to sleep and rapidly I applied a series of continuous sutures to the circular bleeding edge, which stopped the bleeding. After dressing the wound, she was shifted to the ward. My anaesthetist colleague and I stayed with her till next morning. By then she was fully resuscitated and out of danger, but in a state of emotional shock. Since there were no refrigerating facilities available in the hospital, the detached part was washed thoroughly and left in an ice bucket.

We didn't know that the lady was actually the daughter of a very rich and highly influential businessman from India, but realised that when her dad along with his friends and family – accompanied by an entourage of a senior team of top experts in plastic, general and neurosurgery, carrying a box load of dressings, antibiotics, instruments and other surgical accessories – descended on the hospital the next day. Like two junior ministers appearing in front of a Select Committee in a crowded room, my anaesthetist and I presented the clinical story to our guests. I was relieved to hear that none of the expert surgeons present had seen a case of total scalp avulsion before. The party, especially the dad, thanked us profusely. He was pleased to see his daughter alive. The patient was flown back to her hometown a day later. Sadly, the detached scalp had to be thrown away. The last I heard about her was a few months after the accident. At that time she was undergoing cosmetic reconstructive surgery at some European centre of excellence.

I found myself in similar but perhaps more difficult and testing circumstances soon after qualifying as a doctor, just after I had finished twelve months of surgical officer job at the local teaching hospital, which was my only surgical experience at that point in time. I was posted as a Medical Officer at a remote village of Kashmir, in a small dispensary with no surgical facilities. Late in the evening on that eventful day, a full-term pregnant lady who had been in labour at her home for almost two days arrived with her husband, accompanied by a group of male and female villagers. The wise old lady – the *wáren* (midwife) who had managed the patient at home, had advised the family that the baby was already dead in the mother's womb. So, they were seeking help to save the mother and get the dead baby out.

When I heard the story I sent for my two staff colleagues – the healthcare assistant and health visitor who both lived nearby. After examining the patient I could say that it was a breach presentation and I was sure that the baby was still alive – albeit in severe distress. The nearest hospital with obstetric facility was forty miles away and there was no vehicular transport available until the next day afternoon. For the welfare of the mother and the baby the only choice was to perform a Caesarean Section (CS). I knew the steps of this procedure well and had assisted in one before as a final year medical student. The patient would however, need a spinal anaesthetic, which would involve performing a lumbar puncture and injecting the anaesthetic drug into the spinal column to numb the lower half of the body. While I started thinking about the next course of action it occurred to me that I had performed a lumbar puncture once before under supervision and I could administer a spinal anaesthetic. As my thought process gained strength, I suddenly found myself engrossed in an intense mental dilemma about whether or not to undertake the procedure at the dispensary. More than half of me was against the idea of taking such a big risk but I decided to confer with my two helpers. To my utter surprise, both of them were more than keen to proceed. After a brief discussion, unanimously we decided to go ahead.

After explaining the risks and after seeking agreement from the family and the villagers, my two colleagues and I got out all drugs, consumables (such as threads, syringes and gauze) and instruments from various storage areas of the centre. We sterilised these with antiseptics and by boiling. The dispensary dressing room was converted into a makeshift operating room and the examination table into an operating table. With my eyes closed I meditated and prayed for a minute or so, following which I administered the spinal anaesthetic, which luckily did not prove too difficult. With the help of my two eager assistants I performed the Caesarean Section successfully. There were tears and celebrations from everyone inside and outside the makeshift operating theatre when the newly born baby boy cried and inhaled his first breath on earth. We converted the same room into an in-patient bedroom where the mother and child stayed under my care for five days. At the time of discharge both of them were well. The parents left with tears pouring down their eyes. Barely able to control my own emotions, my helpers and I managed to console them and wished all of them well. Soon after they left I went into my little dispensary consultation room, shut the door and had a good cry without anyone noticing it. That was one of the happiest moments of my life.

The scenes described above, that bear semblance to the episodes of the famous 1970 American TV series *MASH*, happened a few decades ago in remote mountainous locales. Since then the world has moved on. Even though healthcare is still in a primitive state in certain parts of the globe, there are now more surgeons, more anaesthetists and more hospitals with better facilities, nicer roads, easily available mechanised transport, and vastly improved communication. Moreover, in today's world patients are highly knowledgeable and better informed.

9

UNUSUAL ENCOUNTERS

Patients bring to us their thoughts and emotions, articulated through words, phrases and sentences, in different forms and styles. Some are vague and longwinded, some are precise and succinct, and some are just one-liners. However, every clinical encounter is a story in itself. Most are forgotten, but a few – even trivial ones – remain implanted on a permanent basis. A colleague remembers an episode during his days as a surgical registrar at a hospital in the North of England, when a Caucasian man in his early twenties was blue lighted into the busy Emergency Department by the ambulance crew in an unconscious state. A few minutes after his arrival, the young fellow started blinking and rolling his eyeballs. As he opened his eyes widely and surveyed the surroundings a couple of times, all of a sudden he sat up and started yelling repeatedly, "Oh, my God! Where am I? Am I in Pakistan?" For a while no one could comprehend why he was saying that. However, it soon dawned on everyone that all clinical personnel standing around the trolley were from South Asian background. He was clearly on the road to recovery.

A surgeon in Saudi Arabia describes a consultation at the end of which he prescribed some tablets to his patient with the aim of reducing the size of his prostate. Whilst he was explaining the therapeutic regime, the patient interrupted him and asked, "Can't you prescribe something that will do both – reduce the size of my prostate and at the same time increase the size of my penis?"

A surgeon from Pakistan was thrown into an ethical dilemma when he was asked, "Sir, I am in a quandary; as you know it's the month of Holy Ramadan and I am fasting. I am thinking of the examination that you just performed on me with your finger through my rear. I am unsure if my fast is still valid? Can you advise me please?"

After a deep thought, the wise clinician replied, "I am a doctor – I mean a surgeon – not an expert on religious affairs, so please do not take my word for it. My view is that if you hated the examination, then the fast is probably intact. If you were okay with it, then your fast is possibly broken." The query might sound trivial or unrelated to the actual illness, but that was something about which the gentleman was most concerned and therefore he wanted an explanation.

A clinical encounter is a two-way street and in order to make an accurate and rapid diagnosis and provide appropriate treatment, the patient must be able to communicate all relevant information about the illness or injury. While sickness can present itself in a deceptive manner with atypical symptoms and signs, a small number of patients withhold information, disclose only half-truths or even try to bend the truth. That can be due to a number of reasons, which include: fear of the unknown, embarrassment, religious or cultural beliefs, family pressures or because they do not wish to present themselves in a negative light. Such clinical scenarios are often tricky and are shrouded in a cloak of secrecy. Separating fiction from fact becomes difficult and it is a challenge for the surgical team to peel away the layers of suspense and expose the factual nucleus without fracturing the mutual bond of trust and understanding with the patient and the family.

THE FEMALE PROSTATE (FROM AM, UK, 2000)

A tall Caucasian blonde lady in her early forties was admitted as an emergency with an overwhelming kidney infection secondary to bilateral obstruction of ureters (tubes connecting the kidneys to urinary bladder) due to compression by a large soft density mass in the pelvis. She stated that in the past she had undergone open abdominal hysterectomy and bilateral oophorectomy (removal of uterus and both ovaries) for uterine fibroids (benign lumps) and since then had been on hormonal replacement therapy. However, there was no abdominal scar present. She did not have any children, and was in a stable relationship with her boyfriend for the last three years. Clinical examination revealed breast implants on both sides. Vaginal examination carried out by a female member of the staff was reported as "difficult and inconclusive".

The lady was examined under anaesthetic (EUA) and cysto-urethroscopy (examination of bladder and water passage) was undertaken at the same time. The findings were bizarre; the urethra was long and there was what appeared like a good size prostate at the bladder-end of the water passage, which was also confirmed on digital rectal examination. The prostate felt benign and blood PSA (prostate specific antigen) reading matched a male of that age. The vagina was obstructed and practically obliterated.

Following the procedure, the lady was interviewed again. This time she broke down and disclosed full facts – she had undergone male to female gender reassignment seven years previously. Penile skin had been inverted to recreate the vagina, which had undergone regular dilatation for a short period thereafter. Her boyfriend was aware of the surgical procedure. The couple never had vaginal intercourse and sexual activity was mostly related to anal sex.

Sadly, after further investigation it became evident that the ureteric obstruction was secondary to advanced cancer arising from the penile skin that had been used to reconstruct the vagina.

Too clean to be true (from NH, UK, 1996)

As the urology registrar on call, I was called to see a Caucasian gentleman in his twenties with injury to his foreskin. The story was odd; he claimed that he had been attacked in a layby by Asian youths who allegedly held him and circumcised him forcefully. However, he did not appear to be shaken by the incident but seemed quite calm and unperturbed. Furthermore, the cut was too clean and not very deep. That raised doubts about the story, but being a grievous racial attack, I told him that the police would have to be involved.

The fear of police involvement instantly brought about a volte-face. He changed his story and confessed that this was a self-inflicted wound that was the result of an act of sexual sadism, which had gone horribly wrong. An urgent psychiatric assessment was arranged, and circumcision was completed under general anaesthetic in the operating theatre.

Beware of a medic! (from SM, UK, 2005)

I was asked to see a GP with the diagnosis of septicaemia secondary to a badly infected scrotum. He was quite vague about the history of events. His initial story was that he had a fall in the bathroom when he sustained injury to his private area. However, he couldn't explain why there was a punctured wound in the scrotum leaking blood and pus.

He became very ill and needed high dependency care for a few days. During that period he became friendly with the nurse looking after him and disclosed to her the factual sequence of events.

He was laying a wooden floor at his home and had hammered a nail through a floorboard into a wooden block when he realised that he had forgotten to adjust one of the other wooden blocks. He released the floorboard that he had just nailed in place but left it turned upside down, with the result that the sharp nail was now pointing upwards. Whilst adjusting the other block he forgot about the nail and as he started moving back on his haunches, he impaled himself on it and it pierced straight into his testicle. He was in agony and for sometime literally nailed to the floor. Somehow he managed to pull himself away. He ended with a small laceration in the scrotum from where dark blood was oozing out. He was too embarrassed about the whole episode and decided not to do anything about it. However, the scrotum started swelling slowly and he developed a large scrotal hematoma (collection of blood), which subsequently became infected. He continued to treat himself at home with oral antibiotics, but in the end became desperate and had no choice except to come to the hospital.

IDENTITY CRISIS (FROM TH, INDIA, 1995)

This bizarre case was discussed in our weekly clinical meeting during my surgical training days. A young man in his thirties from a nearby village who worked in the local animal husbandry department attended the surgical department for investigation of primary infertility. As part of the investigation the consultant-in-charge arranged semen analysis. A couple of hours after the patient handed over the semen specimen to the laboratory, the technician contacted the pathologist for urgent help to review the slides, because he was seeing some "weird looking objects" under the microscope.

The pathologist had a look at the slides and found bizarre shapes that did not look like normal human sperms. He could not come to any conclusion and the next day he explained to the patient that the sample of semen was probably not collected or preserved properly. He advised him to provide a new sample. On hearing this, the patient became disturbed and refused to provide a sample straightaway. However, after persuasion, he promised to bring one in later.

A new sample was submitted, which was as weird as the first one. The pathologist had never seen sperms of that shape and size before. In the next one-on-one meeting the pathologist informed the patient that a semen analysis report could not be issued. On hearing that the patient became shaky and tearful and begged the doctor to issue a report. "If I am not able to prove to my in-laws that I am fertile, my marriage will break up," he pleaded. When asked about the reasons for that, he revealed the truth.

He admitted that he had been investigated for infertility a few years before after his first marriage and had several semen tests done, all of which had shown absence of sperms. That had in fact been the main reason for the break-up of his first marriage. Subsequently he had remarried but had not disclosed to his new wife or in-laws anything about his fertility status. After a couple of years of wedlock he was pressed by his second wife and her parents to get himself investigated.

Finding himself in a tight corner, he pinched a semen specimen from his work place – courtesy of a technician friend who was working in the artificial insemination unit. It became clear that the "weird looking objects" were sperms that belonged to a bull and not a human.

It follows that, when it comes to your health, disclosure of factual information makes things easier for the provider as well as the recipient of care. However, being overzealously open or outspoken can sometimes throw the clinician off the rails. Like a stage actor who forgets the pre-rehearsed script, the clinician has to adjust the bearings quickly and ensure that the show carries on.

HONESTY – THE BEST POLICY! (FROM PS, UK, 2002)

Many years ago I was asked by a legal firm to provide a medico-legal report on a man in his thirties. He had been involved in a road traffic accident a few months before and suffered from the after effects of back injury that he had sustained.

Dressed smartly in a blue jacket, grey trousers and freshly polished black shoes the handsome young man greeted me with a firm handshake. As a matter of routine I asked him, "What do you do for a living, my friend?"

"I steal cars," he replied unhesitatingly.

I looked at him in disbelief. My facial appearance must have been sufficiently alarming since he commented immediately, "Doctor, I am not joking, I have actually been honest with you." Emphasising the point further he added, "I am a car thief, but don't worry, your car is absolutely safe!"

NERVOUS NELLIE (FROM SK, UK, 1998)

A young lady in her thirties who was a highflier in the world of banking and finance and worked in the City of London, was due to undergo nephrectomy (kidney removal) for localised kidney cancer. She arrived on the ward on the morning of surgery and was agitated and nervous about the impending surgical procedure. She said to the ward staff that she was not scared of the operation and had total confidence in the surgeon and the hospital, but she was worried about the blood transfusion, and wanted a guarantee that no blood would be administered to her whilst she was under anaesthetic. However, she was unwilling to disclose the reasons for her anxiety to anyone other than the operating surgeon.

The news was relayed to me in theatre. So I went to see her on the ward and found her in a fidgety state. I started the conversation by asking, "Mrs R, I hear that you do not wish to have a blood transfusion. Are you a Jehovah's Witness?"

"No, no, I am not but I do not want any blood transfusion and I need assurance from you regarding this before you operate on me," she said in a commanding tone.

"Why is that?" I asked curiously.

In a muffled voice she replied, "It may sound silly, Mr K, but I do not want other people to hear what I am about to say."

"Okay. Let's go to sister's office and have a chat," I said reassuringly.

Continuing the conversation in a hushed tone she asked, "If you transfused blood to me, would you know who the blood donor was? You wouldn't – would you?"

"No, but the donor is tested thoroughly before being bled," I explained.

"Well, that might be so, but the donor could be anyone – a prostitute, a drug user or for that matter anyone, even any coloured man or woman – I mean a non-Caucasian person. I refuse to have the blood of such persons transfused into me," she declared.

I was taken aback and could not figure out how to respond. The problem for me was not about what she had said, but she was saying that to me – her surgeon, who was a non-Caucasian. However, before I could respond, perhaps realising her mistake she added, "Please don't get me wrong – I really trust you."

After a careful pause I responded assertively, "Thank you for that, but if you really trust me then you ought to stop worrying about the things that you just mentioned. If a blood transfusion will be required to save your life then you will have one."

She did not argue any further. Thankfully, the operation went well and no blood transfusion was required.

BLESSING IN DISGUISE (FROM BC, UK, 2000)

I undertook radical prostatectomy for cancer of prostate on Mr D – a sixty-five-year-old business executive. Accompanied by his elegant and smartly dressed wife in her early fifties, the patient returned for follow-up consultation a few months after the operation. As always, the wife did most of the talking. At the conclusion of the consultation, I advised the patient to return in four months for another consultation following a blood test a week before the appointment. At this point the patient's wife started the conversation, which went something like this:

"It is great, Mr C – my husband is cancer free – he has no urinary leakage, no pain, and our sex life is great and that is a bonus."

"I am very pleased to hear that, Mrs D," I replied with a smile.

"I would like to tell you something else – you know in a Hollywood film they never tell you the real thing about something that we women often talk about."

"And what is that?" I asked curiously.

"The first thing a lady will do after sex is go to the washroom. But they never show that. Do they? We women call it the sticky legs syndrome or the wet patch syndrome."

My clinic nurse and I just looked at each other and did not quite know how to react. The conversation was becoming embarrassing and we both were feeling uneasy. I decided not to respond to her comment, but before I could say anything, she continued, "You see I do not have to suffer from this any more!"

Initially I didn't quite understand why she was telling me all that but soon the penny dropped. What Mrs D was actually saying was that as a consequence of the surgical operation Mr D was not able to ejaculate.

I had to say something and therefore I muttered, "Well, that is an inevitable consequence of this procedure, Mrs D, do you remember I explained to you the reasons for that before your husband had the operation?"

However, without paying attention to my remark she carried on, "And not only this, Mr C, oral sex is fantastic now, as there is nothing to swallow any more! Thank you so much. We will see you in four months."

As Mr and Mrs D left the consultation room – smilingly holding each other's hands – the clinic nurse and I took deep sighs in disbelief. It took us a few minutes to recover before we could call our next patient.

CASH & CARRY (FROM KT, INDIA 1970)

Many decades ago I used to work as a general surgeon in a Christian Missionary hospital in India. It was a Friday morning – my regular outpatient clinic day. There was no appointment system but the clinic was always overcrowded and the workload always exceeded capacity.

A pretty girl in her late teens, walking with a limp, came into the room. An older man probably in his fifties with a large cream coloured turban on his head introduced himself as her uncle. The girl had a sinus (a small hole) below the knee that was discharging thick creamy pus. She suffered from osteomyelitis (infection of bone) of tibia (leg bone) and needed a sequestrectomy (removal of dead bone), which used to be a common surgical operation in those days.

As they started leaving the room, I captured a fleeting glance of the man's back and noticed a large hump protruding from below the nape of his neck. Was he carrying an object of that shape or was it something attached to his body? Since I was overwhelmed by a mass of patients who were to be seen in a short space of time I did not bother to investigate, and within a couple of minutes I forgot about it.

The outpatient clinic finished at around 2pm. I left the building and started walking through the hospital gardens towards the inpatient wing and saw the young girl basking in the warm autumn sunshine on the grassy lawn nearby. The girl greeted me with a shy smile. Her uncle was sitting nearby and was absorbed in his own thoughts. As I walked past, I remembered the hump that I had seen earlier. My curiosity made me walk back towards the man. I could see the hump and therefore asked if I could examine him in the clinic room nearby, to which he agreed readily.

As he made himself comfortable on a stool, he reminded me gently that he had only come to the hospital to get his niece treated and that he was not interested in his own treatment. However, he did not object to my examination, which revealed a lipoma (fatty lump) of the size of a large watermelon, about two kilograms in weight, sitting on a rather narrow base just below the nape of his neck. Whilst I was examining him he told me that he'd had this lump for many years and that he was not bothered about it.

After washing my hands I said to him, "It is quite a weight hanging on your back. It must be difficult for you to manage. I will be quite happy to remove it for you by a surgical operation."

"It is not giving me any problem, but err... err... if you say so, sir – but..."

"But what?" I interrupted.

"What I was saying is that if you remove this, how much will you pay me?" he said hesitatingly.

I was taken aback by his response, but managed to hide my discomfiture. As I started to speak he interjected, "Sir, you are a wise man, look at the size of the thing and then decide how much." He was clearly inviting me to give him a figure and was trying to negotiate the best price.

Smilingly I replied, "I will think about that and let you know."

I saw him many times over the next few weeks during the course of his niece's treatment. Even though my hands itched to take the lump off his back, neither he nor I raised the subject again.

THE MISSING HAIRCLIP (FROM MK, UK, 2001)

The incident happened during the first year of my appointment as a consultant. A young lad of sixteen returned to Emergency Department complaining of abdominal pain; he had been operated for appendicectomy by my registrar two weeks before. His grandfather – a retired British army surgeon accompanied him.

The registrar on duty, who had not been involved with his care on his previous admission, attended the call. During the consultation the army surgeon gave the registrar a hard time and lectured him about how good things used to be during his days as a surgeon, particularly in the armed forces. He also wanted explanations for his grandson's continuing symptoms. The apologetic registrar listened attentively and arranged an abdominal x-ray, which embarrassingly revealed a hair clip lodged in the patient's pelvis. That worked like fuel to a fire – the old lion became furious and started blaming the hospital. The registrar could not take the wrath any more, so he rang me for help, and after hearing the story I decided to see the patient.

As I entered the cubicle, without any introductions, the retired surgeon – dressed in a double-breasted blazer with sharply creased trousers – started having a go at me. "That is the problem, the clip must have fallen into the wound at the time of the operation. I am going to be honest with you; I am going to make sure that the hospital, you – and I mean you all – are made to pay for this gross error."

I did not respond to his comments straightaway, but felt overwhelmed. After examining the patient I looked at the x-ray and then said, "Sir, to me it seems unlikely that a hairclip belonging to a female scrub nurse would have dropped into the open wound at the time of the operation without anyone noticing it. However, as you yourself know, anything is possible in surgery…"

The old hat continued with his barrage with an air of authority; he was simply not prepared to listen. At the end of an unhelpful conversation I said, "I suggest that we take your grandson to theatre for examination under anaesthetic. Should you wish to do so, I have no objection to you coming to theatre whilst I examine and re-explore your grandson's abdomen under anaesthetic."

He agreed to my suggestion but continued to tell me how disciplined things used to be during his time as an army surgeon.

After the patient was anaesthetised, I put my gloved right

forefinger into the patient's rectum and retrieved the missing hair clip. Involuntarily I said, "Here we are, sir! Have you got an explanation how this hairclip went there?" Without any further word, like a dog with his tail tucked between his hind legs, the old master left the scene.

When the youngster was asked later about what had actually happened, he admitted that he had been playing with his friend at home who inserted the clip into his rectum, and when they tried to retrieve it, they couldn't.

Finding weird objects inside human bodies is not uncommon in surgical practice. In many cases there is a psychiatric reason for the deviant activity. A surgical colleague recalls managing a patient who was admitted to the hospital after having ingested metallic nails. He was put on observation for the night. The next morning, the curtain around the hospital bed was found on the floor. It emerged that the metal hooks holding the curtain were missing. These were subsequently found lying in his stomach.

The problem can occasionally arise out of sheer ignorance. A clinician from Ireland recalls removing a thermometer from a young lady's bladder under general anaesthetic. As part of the infertility management she had been advised to chart her basal temperature using a digital basal thermometer, which is more sensitive than a normal thermometer for recording minor temperature fluctuations. Her explanation was that basal temperature meant temperature of the base. When asked to clarify what she meant by base, she replied, *'the hot seat where all the activity takes place.'* So, every morning she would insert the thermometer into her vagina and measure the temperature. That day, after insertion, the thermometer disappeared, and neither her husband nor she could find it. She had actually introduced the end of the thermometer into her urethra, and as she pushed it further the device slipped into her bladder.

In the majority of cases, however, the principal objective of introducing objects is sexual fantasy, but when things go wrong, help is needed. A colleague recounts a case when a vibrator had jammed in the rectum and was still vibrating when the patient attended the Emergency Department. Another clinician had to look after a patient who had inserted an Internet connecting cable through the penile opening with the intention of 'getting online', and the prongs were stuck in the mid-urethra.

The surgical literature is actually full of bizarre reports of a similar nature, but here is an anecdote from my own memory bank when an unusual object was retrieved in unusual circumstances.

As the urology registrar on call, I was asked to see a recently married accountant from Asian background in his thirties who had presented with acute retention of urine and urethral pain. The patient was in obvious discomfort and in a panic state – shaking and sweating. I tried to calm him down and as the nurse went out, and he and I were alone in the cubicle, hurriedly he sat up and said, "Doctor, I need to tell you something in confidence before the nurse comes back. My wife is in New York, in connection with her work, so I was alone at home. I don't know how to say this – um, um, I started playing with myself – I know I shouldn't have done that but I did. I got a golden bangle from my wife's jewellery box – one that straightens on opening. I inserted it into my water passage, through my thingy. As I pushed it the damn thing disappeared inside. What am I going to do? My marriage is finished. Please don't tell anyone that I told you that. And please, please do not tell my wife or my family – I will be dead if she finds out and I will mess up my marriage and lose my family."

I calmed him down and after admitting him to the hospital, took him to theatre and examined him under general anaesthetic. The straightened bangle was lying snugly in the urethra along its curvature. Luckily, it could be retrieved without much difficulty because the proximal end was not very far from the external urinary opening. After he regained consciousness I handed it over to him personally. He was discharged home on the same day.

The gentleman returned for follow-up after a couple of weeks. On this occasion he was a completely different person – elegantly dressed, confident and chirpy. He was totally pain free and was passing urine very well. As he was about to leave I asked him, "What did you tell your wife?"

"Actually, I didn't tell her anything. She does not even know that I was in the hospital and had an operation – you know she was out of the country. I also requested my GP not to disclose it to her." And with a big laugh he added, "I am pleased that the thing is safely back in her jewellery box – you know doctor, the thing is twenty-two carat gold and is worth a bob or two."

"I bet it is," I replied.

Some patients bring with them their own solutions to get round minor technical issues – like fixing a catheter or a catheter bag to the thigh or leg, stopping a urostomy or colostomy bag from leaking, fixing a surgical dressing securely, and so on. Some of the ideas are novel and interesting but experimentation can sometimes create difficulties for the individual, and when things go wrong, for whatever reason, surgical help becomes necessary.

DIGGING FOR GOLD (FROM TV, UK, 1973)

The incident happened during the course of my training in urology, before the era of self-lubricating catheters and fibre optics. A mechanic in his late thirties attended the hospital at periodic intervals for dilatation of a terminal urethral stricture for which he required sedation. After a few sessions he decided to practise self-dilatation using a self-designed oval, tapering gold plated ear stud screwed on at the narrow end to a slightly flexible fibreglass rod. He preferred this rather than coming regularly to the hospital. He used to sterilise the contraption by boiling and cooling it.

During one of the self-dilatation sessions, the gold plated

metal stud got disconnected from the shaft and was lost in his bladder. It was removed with great difficulty with a rigid cystoscope under general anaesthetic.

A FISHY BUSINESS (FROM RB, ZIMBABWE, 1994)

I was working as a surgeon at a hospital in Rhodesia (present day Zimbabwe). A non-white African man in his fifties was admitted with vague complaints of feeling unwell. On further questioning he said, "I have a fish in my bladder." The patient had been treated previously for a urethral stricture. Because he lived in a remote village miles away from the hospital, on discharge he had been given a metal bougie (dilator) with instructions about how to self-dilate his urethral stricture. However, he misplaced the instrument, but he noted that the local river fish was of the same calibre and length as the metal dilator. So he caught a fish and negotiated it into the urethra. Unfortunately while the fish could be introduced down the urethra, due to the direction of the scales it could not be withdrawn, and so it ended up in his urethra and bladder. The dead fish had to be removed by an open operation. Literature search revealed similar cases of fish in the bladder reported by others, but in all of them the fish had actively swum into the bladder.

BOTTLED UP (FROM TH, SRI LANKA, 1992)

I was working as a registrar in surgery. A lady in her late seventies came to the clinic along with her husband of the same age, complaining of painful rectal prolapse. This was reduced easily in front of the husband without the need of a general anaesthetic. She was advised surgery as a means of permanent cure. The risks of the proposed operation were explained.

However, the couple declined having any surgical intervention.

More than one year later the couple returned again in a distressed and embarrassed state. The lady complained of abdominal pain and the conversation with the husband was something like the following:

"I am utterly ashamed to tell you what happened. My wife had the red ball coming out of her back passage. I used to push it back myself, initially with my hand, but as it became bigger I used a coke bottle base to push it back. That used to work fine and with time the whole bottle started going in, but I was always able to retrieve it. This time I couldn't."

Examination and subsequent x-ray revealed that the bottle had migrated upwards and was sitting in the lower part of colon. It was removed without much difficulty. On this occasion, however, she agreed to have the operative procedure.

Some clinical scenarios are not only awkward, but they pose an ethical dilemma for the surgeon, who by the very nature of the job is in a position of responsibility to bring the issue to a satisfactory endpoint. In some cases, diplomacy and wisdom are required to resolve a difficult and often sensitive matter.

At the very dawn of my surgical training in India, an illiterate labourer in his thirties and his wife of a similar age presented at the teaching hospital for advice. The wife had developed a lump in the abdomen, for which she had seen a local quack. He had hinted to the family that she might be pregnant. The couple had five children; the oldest was eight years old. The husband had undergone a vasectomy by one of the surgical residents at the same hospital about one year before.

On clinical examination it was obvious that the lady was pregnant, with gestational age of about twenty-four weeks. However, as soon as the boss declared the diagnosis to the couple, the husband started abusing the wife and accusing her of being unfaithful and the wife was blaming the hospital by saying that her husband's operation had not been done properly. Whilst the couple were arguing intensely, the boss, who was normally a man of very few words, interrupted by saying, "Stop shouting," and addressing the husband he added, "Look, we will settle this issue by getting your semen tested."

A week later the couple, accompanied by their two youngest children, a few older ladies and a large number of village elders, arrived together to find out the result of semen analysis. The laboratory report had revealed azoospermia (absence of sperms), which meant that the operation had been successful. On seeing the result the boss took a deep breath and said to the lady, "Can I please examine you again?"

He took her into the next room and whilst she lay on the couch behind the curtained barrier, he asked her husband and her companions to stay outside, and in the presence of the nursing and medical staff questioned her about a range of matters such as the details of the family, sources of income and social background. It was clear that they had an impoverished upbringing and the story about her being pregnant following her husband's vasectomy had not only disseminated to their neighbourhood, but to the entire locality where they lived. She had become the talk of the whole village and everyone was curious to know the result of the semen test.

After musing for a while, the boss looked around and said to the lady, "I am going to save you and your children this time, but only if you promise me not to commit the mistake again."

Without any hesitation she whispered back, " I promise you, sir, but please save me."

The boss returned to his chair, called all her relatives into the room and after taking a deep breath started addressing them, "There is no doubt that she is pregnant. However, the semen test result shows that the vasectomy operation was not performed properly. The problem is that the doctor who performed the operation does not work at this hospital any more; he went abroad for higher studies."

There were scenes of jubilation all round. The family and the village elders started celebrating, hugging and congratulating one another. The medical and nursing staff were stunned.

When the crowd left, the boss sighed again, removed his glasses, rubbed his face and with a tired look in his eyes lifted up his head and said, "Right or wrong, I did it for the young family," and after a period of silence he added, "Do you know, they would have lynched her if I hadn't done what I did." After a further pause the old master concluded, "Have you heard of the English proverb: 'maternity is a matter of fact, paternity is a matter of opinion'." I didn't know then that it is an American and not an English proverb.

The episode happened more than four decades ago in the Eastern hemisphere within a small community where there was a clear risk of the subject being punished in public. In similar circumstances, would every clinician have thought it ethically right to deviate from the truth for the larger good of the patient and the family, and if it emerged that he had lied, how would the patient's family and the larger society judge him?

By its very nature, a clinical encounter exposes the private life of an individual to external scrutiny and occasionally important issues like morality and confidentiality are brought into focus. However, those seeking clinical advice should not be restrained by the fear that their medical condition or personal circumstances will become public knowledge. The rules of conduct haven't changed over the years but have been fine-tuned to remain fit for purpose. The 2013 GMC document 'Good Medical Practice', which is the code of practice for clinicians in the UK stipulates that, '*you must not express your personal beliefs (including political, religious and moral beliefs) to patients in ways that exploit their vulnerability or are likely to cause them distress*' – words not very different from what Hippocrates advised us centuries ago. Mutual trust and confidentiality of information are in fact enshrined in the Hippocratic Oath, which stipulates that, '*I will respect the privacy of my patients, for their problems are not disclosed to me that the world may know…"* (modern version). The classical (original) version of the Oath written nearly 2500 years ago used the phrase, *"keep sacred and secret within my own breast.'* And that is what the three colleagues did in their respective circumstances.

THE DARK SECRET (FROM SR, UK, 1996)

During my tenure as a registrar I was asked to see Mr T, a city executive in his early forties, who was accompanied by his wife of similar age and a young daughter in her late teens. The patient complained of severe pain in the urethra and was also bleeding per urethra. The story given to me was that he had arrived home early from work in the afternoon and as the day progressed, his symptoms had worsened. When his family returned home, they decided to bring him to the hospital.

I admitted the patient to the ward and told the family that the cause of his symptoms needed to be investigated. After his family had left, the patient disclosed to me that he had not been at work all day; instead he had been with his mistress. They were playing games and she had inserted a hatpin into his urethra that couldn't be retrieved. The more she tried, the more painful it became, and it then started bleeding. Mr T also told me to keep the information secret.

I made arrangements to take Mr T to the operating theatre to remove the foreign body under general anaesthetic. The pin was stuck into the wall of the urethra (water passage) and was removed with little difficulty.

Whilst I was in theatre, his wife had rung the ward and on hearing that her husband had been taken to the operating theatre, she and the daughter rushed back to the hospital. As I was leaving they confronted me at the theatre entrance. "What was the problem with my husband?" the wife asked me nervously.

I had to make an instant decision about what to say. "Actually, after you left I decided to take him to theatre to stop the bleeding. I am pleased to say that he is perfectly fine now. He was bleeding from a blood vessel."

"Thank goodness, we are so grateful to you," she replied.

The patient was discharged home next morning and never returned. His secret remained safe.

LIGHTNING STRIKES TWICE (FROM PS, UK, 2000)

The bizarre incident happened when I was working as a registrar at a London teaching hospital. I was called to the Emergency Department to see Mr J – a man in his early fifties, who was accompanied by a lady of similar age. He complained of penile pain and swelling. After listening to the history and after examination, it emerged that he had sustained a fracture of the penis. This usually happens due to physical injury to a fully erect penis during sexual activity and leads to sudden loss of erection, extensive bruising and painful swelling of the penis.

The gentleman lived in the North of England and on a visit to London that day, he had run into the lady who had been his girlfriend more than twenty years previously. One thing had led to another and the two ended up in her flat and during their passionate sexual encounter he sustained a penile fracture.

Notwithstanding the fact that penile fracture is a rare condition, surprisingly both of them knew the diagnosis. That made me inquisitive and I asked Mr J, "This is not a very common diagnosis, but you seem to know all about it."

"Yes, I do. The thick sheet that covers the erectile tissue of the penis splits if the erect penis is handled roughly," he said.

"Yes, that is correct, but how do you know all that?" I asked.

"I read about it."

That made me even more curious and I asked, "But why did you read about such a rare condition?"

"I do not know how to say this doctor… you will not believe it; this is actually the second time. The truth is that I sustained a fracture of my penis twenty years ago."

And at this point the lady interjected, "And on that occasion, like today, I was responsible for putting him through pain. It is unbelievable that the same thing happened with us twice – sorry but I am being honest with you, I feel so guilty."

Continuing the conversation the patient added, "We were friends then. Today's meeting was just a chance; I met her at the underground station after a span of almost twenty years. I never expected to see her again after such a long time. I guess we both got carried away. We should have been careful but please keep it a secret." He tried to explain and after a pause added, "I guess it will need to be repaired surgically – like last time? When will I be discharged from the hospital, doctor?"

"Hopefully tomorrow," I replied.

"That is okay, I can make an excuse for tonight," he said, appearing more concerned about his return journey home than his physical predicament.

A NOD AND A SMILE (FROM PT, UK, 1996)

Mr C underwent resection for a large prostate at a London teaching hospital where I was working as a registrar. The family were Jehovah's witnesses and were therefore insistent that no blood or blood products were to be administered before, during or after the operation.

As the procedure progressed, Mr C started bleeding profusely from the prostatic bed leading to a significant blood loss. Worse still, the patient continued to bleed in the recovery area, resulting in a drop in haemoglobin from the preoperative level of 130G/L to 70G/L.

It was decided to take Mr C back to theatre to have a second look and try to locate the bleeding points. However, after trying for about an hour, apart from generalised ooze from the prostatic cavity, no major bleeder was identified, but by then his haemoglobin level had dropped further to 50G/L.

A large number of family members came to visit Mr C that evening. They were advised about the dire necessity of blood transfusion for Mr C. The request was rejected flatly. In fact they were annoyed that we had raised the subject with them and left the hospital in the evening saying that they would organise a prayer meeting at the community centre.

Mr C's clinical condition continued to deteriorate further. Even though the bleeding had somewhat eased, the haemoglobin level continued to fall and he became short of breath and was quite poorly. Being the registrar on call for the night I was called to see him late in the evening and while I was alone with the patient in the side ward where he was being nursed he said to me, "Doctor, I don't want to die."

"Mr C, you need a blood transfusion but you and your family do not want that."

"Can you give me some blood but keep that a secret, and please, please do not disclose that to my family."

Immediately I arranged four units of blood and transfused three of these to him overnight. I made sure that the family did not know anything about the transfusion. By next morning he had improved markedly and was sitting up in bed.

The family arrived in the morning and as I met them in the corridor Mr C's brother said to me, "Doc, he looks so well; what do you say now?"

I shook his hand, and with a nod and a broad smile said, "Yes, he does look better," and walked down the corridor.

Some encounters are not only strange and unexpected, but also have a sweet and innocent flavour and reflect kindness and decency .

Remember me (FROM DC, CARIBBEAN, 2000)

As fourth year medical students in the West Indies, we were keen to practise physical examination on patients. Whenever we discovered patients with classic or interesting signs, we would spread the word around which would be something like: There is a man with a lipoma (benign fatty tumour) on bed twenty-one on victory ward; or there is a palpable kidney on bed five on patience ward; or there is an interesting thyroid on bed ten on emergency surgical ward, and so on.

I became a junior surgical resident at the same hospital where I trained as a medical student. On my way to the outpatient clinic, along the crowded hospital corridor, a young woman smiled at me, started walking by my side and then said, "Do you remember me? You saw me two years ago when I was admitted to the hospital."

Hesitatingly I replied, "Um, you look familiar... but sorry, I cannot recollect. Anyway, how are you doing now?"

"Try to remember me, doc, I am the 'spleen on bed four' who was admitted to surgical ward!"

Suddenly the penny dropped, "Oh, yes, I do remember you, but what are you doing here today?" I asked.

"I have been invited to take part in the MBBS examinations for doctors. I hope they all pass this time," she said with a chuckle.

The young lady had an enlarged spleen that had been felt by hundreds of medical students, examiners as well as examinees, including me.

Last wish (FROM AM, IRAN, 1984)

I was working as a general surgeon at a small hospital in a remote town in the Kurdistan Province in Iran. One evening I was called to see a very sick patient in his sixties, who was markedly emaciated and dehydrated, and complained of difficulty in swallowing for many months. This had worsened over a period of time, making it difficult for him to swallow even liquids. I made a provisional diagnosis of cancer of oesophagus (food pipe), which was quite common in that part of the world. However, there were very few facilities available locally to treat.

The patient was unwilling to travel to a bigger centre and wanted to be cared for locally. After hydrating him with intravenous fluids, under local anaesthetic I made a hole in his stomach and inserted a Malecot's catheter (a rubber tube with a self expanding end), so that he could feed himself through the tube without having to eat and swallow. The operation is known as gastrostomy.

Following the procedure, everything started working well for him; he was quite happy to be able to feed himself through the tube. I arranged for a follow-up appointment in two months time, but in my mind I doubted if he would survive that long. To my surprise and delight he returned looking much better. I even started wondering whether my diagnosis of cancer was correct. However, when I asked him to drink water it was clear the disease had progressed to the point that he was unable to swallow anything – not even water. Once again I advised referral to a specialised centre, which was about 200 miles away, but again he declined. Instead he requested for the tube to be replaced by a larger one, so that he could enjoy his food more. Not withstanding his son's comment, "Sir, please do not agree to everything he says; do you know he was telling me to ask you to implant a denture to his stomach tube," I complied with his request.

One month later I met the son in the local main street. He told me that his dad had passed away. On his deathbed, however, he had insisted that the stomach tube that had given him a new lease of life for many months be buried along with him. I was surprised to know that the family had complied with his request.

MAN'S BEST FRIEND
(FROM SR, REPUBLIC OF IRELAND, 2008)

This was the first year of my consultant career. Accompanied by my team I went to see Mr D, a middle-aged builder on whom I had performed left nephrectomy for kidney cancer the previous day. He appeared very cheerful and was sitting in a chair by his bed. As I started talking to him, through the corner of my eye on his side desk I noticed the picture of a German shepherd dog with a greeting card in front of it that read, "Sam, thank you for saving my life." I was too embarrassed to ask why he was thanking the dog and not me.

Two days later I saw him again; by now he was ready to be discharged, and I finally gathered the nerve to ask the question, "Who is Sam and how did he save your life Mr D…?"

"Actually, Mr R, my dog Sam jumped at me and pushed me with the result that I landed heavily on the left side of my back. I had to attend the hospital with marked pain in my left loin. They suspected that I had damaged my kidney but the scan showed a big tumour sitting in my left kidney. If he hadn't pushed me, we wouldn't have known that. Would we?"

In summary clinicians are incredibly lucky to meet, greet and treat people from every spectre of society. They come to see us to talk about their troubles. In the process they communicate their apprehensions and worries, disclose their sensitive secrets, brood over their disappointments and share their joys. In a nutshell, they open their hearts and minds to us. Each encounter however trivial or tricky, concise or complicated, is a journey into the multi-coloured landscape of human psyche and makes us better prepared for the next one waiting in the queue. While some situations pose challenges, they also make the working life of a clinician varied and interesting. The maxims: 'there is no end to learning', and 'experience is the father of wisdom' apply befittingly to the world of surgery.

10

COMMUNICATION

Communication is defined as the act of imparting or exchanging information by speaking, writing, or using some other medium. It is a dynamic process by which the information is transferred to create a shared understanding between the sender and the receiver. Communication can be verbal or non-verbal. Verbal communication is the act of expressing one's thoughts in words. A huge amount of that is in the form of spoken words. The vast majority of doctors, in particular surgeons, are articulate communicators and complement their spoken words with non-verbal body language that is appropriate for the occasion. A small minority exhibit persuasive eloquence, particularly when in action on the frontline – like Mr K who was one of my bosses during my training days.

Mr K received patients from all over the world. He undertook complex procedures, sometimes spending a whole day for a single case. Seeing him at work was like watching an accomplished sculptor carving an object of imagination. He was normally quiet and reserved but as soon as he touched a patient in the operating theatre, his personality would suddenly transform into a chatterbox and he would start a non-stop monologue. It was as if the sterile theatre gear acted as an on and off switch that triggered his speech centre. The topics were varied and included travel, history, films, stocks and shares, politics, gardening and, of course surgery. Usually there would be visitors in theatre watching the maestro at work who had no other option but to listen to him. If there was nobody there, the chatter would still continue and the person at the receiving end would be his regular anaesthetist. Seated on a stool at the head end of the operating table behind a curtained barrier he would occasionally respond with phrases such as: 'really'; 'how interesting'; 'that is extraordinary' or simply with interjections and fillers like 'uh, um, uh-huh, hmm, ah' and so on. I guess over the years he too had become conditioned to a routine.

I also remember a colleague about whom it was well known that he shouldn't be disturbed while he was operating. The theatre sister would signal a warning to everyone, "Please don't speak to him now, we have got to finish this list." The anaesthetist and other permanent staff had also learnt not to speak to him whilst he was tied up. If he asked a question, the respondent would normally reply with a single word or in short phrases to avoid a conversation. The issue was that if anyone started a dialogue with him he would put down his tools and begin narrating a long story whilst everyone waited and while the anaesthetised patient laid on the table. He would either blow his own trumpet in the form of a protracted discourse about his experiences "during the good old days", or describe in fine detail a case that he had seen before.

Worse still is to cope with a surgeon who is a habitual chatterer but who repeats the same talk time and time again. To be at the receiving end of such an individual can be a nightmare.

My hairdresser (from Co, Republic of Ireland, 2001)

Mr O was well known for his exuberantly chatty nature and had the habit of injecting humour into a conversation – perhaps too often! He was particularly known for his cryptic jokes, each of which would generate three episodes of laughter: first when he blurted out the joke loudly, which would be accompanied by an equally loud paroxysm of laughter from him. As a matter of courtesy the audience also tried to laugh with him. This would be followed by a second chuckle by everyone (except him) after the joke actually sank in. Finally the audience would complete the sequence with independent sheepish giggles for the absurdity or sometimes the lack of humour in the joke.

I was the anaesthetist for Mr O's theatre list for that afternoon and saw Mr Z – one of Mr O's regular patients, on my pre-anaesthetic ward round. As I was about to leave his bedside he stopped me and said, "Doctor, can I ask you a favour? I see a new anaesthetist every time I come in for this procedure and I make the same request each time. Can you put me to sleep please? I do not want a spinal or local anaesthetic."

"Is there a reason for that, Mr Z?" I asked curiously.

Hesitatingly he replied, "Umm … doctor, yes there is; I have been under Mr O for a few years. You know how he is – a bit like my regular hairdresser Bob. Whenever Bob touches my hair he starts talking and doesn't stop until he finishes, and every time he talks about only one thing – football. Likewise, whenever Mr O touches me he starts talking. Whilst I am lying on the table fully awake, Mr O carries on non-stop with his silly jokes. I can't stand these any more because I have heard them so many times. Don't tell him, but they are not amusing either."

Conversely, some characters are capable of inflicting neurological damage on their juniors by muttering a single phrase or a sentence, like: "Young lady, cerebrate before you phonate!" Some do that simply by pressing the mute button.

The silent treatment (*from JT, Pakistan, 1984*)

During my surgical residency I worked for Professor S who was very well known since he had left surgical scars on some of the elite of civil society in my part of the world. His once-weekly ward round used to be the highlight of the departmental timetable. Residents would get ready for the event by preparing cases for presentation, which were allocated to them by the second-in-command.

Professor S was not only a man of very few words but he was also an expert in responding to a question with a question, with the result that very few people mustered the courage to ask him a question. Sustained silence was his ultimate weapon.

One day a young and confident colleague of mine – also a junior resident, started presenting a patient who had been admitted the night before after having been hit in the abdomen by a bull. At the very start of the presentation Professor S's silent and penetrating look locked on to the resident who suddenly fell to pieces.

"Sir, this patient was hit by err... err... err..." she struggled.

The boss stayed still and did not say anything. So the resident started again. "Sir, he was hit by err... err, what you call, a err... err..."

None of the fifteen or so people standing around the bed, including me, had the courage to prompt the word 'bull' to the victim in distress. It all became rather embarrassing but there was absolutely no change in Professor S's facial configuration or posture. The resident who was by now pale and sweaty had another go and said, "Sir, this man was admitted last night after being hit on the abdomen by the husband of a cow." There was a roar of laughter – with the exception of Professor S who did not even flicker.

Sometimes clinicians are consumed in their own thoughts and forget the central character – the patient. An orthopaedic colleague described an incident when his boss was doing a knee arthroscopy (looking inside a joint with a telescope). Without realising that the procedure was being performed under a spinal anaesthetic and the patient was awake, he muttered the words, "That joint looks rotten." A couple of minutes later the anaesthetist started getting concerned because the patient's oxygen saturation was falling. Fortunately he recovered and the surgeon had to apologise.

In 2010 the UK Department of Health and the NHS Institute of Innovation and Improvement (III) commissioned King's College London and The King's Fund to undertake research into what matters most to patients? Unsurprisingly the respondents stated that experience of care was as important to them as clinical safety and effectiveness. The Care Quality Commission (CQC) – the UK's health and social care regulator considers patient experience as one of the important domains of the regulatory framework and healthcare providers are assessed by the results of patient questionnaire surveys. One of the important questions in the survey is: "Did doctors talk in front of you as if you weren't there?" The sad fact (according to CQC statistics) is that about one in four patients think that they do.

Talking in front of patients as if they aren't there implies that they are of no consequence. The truth is that they are the purpose and usually the focus of the conversation. I believe it is a habit that feeds into clinical behaviour from medical student days after one watches peers, teachers and bosses in action. I have witnessed it innumerable times, and have been sometimes guilty of it myself without even knowing about it. Like any bad habit, controlling it is an active process that needs a conscious effort. The worst scenario is when while talking over a patient one uses a word or a phrase that is misunderstood.

COLLATERAL DAMAGE (FROM JL, UK, *1986*)

The incident happened when I was working as a registrar in surgery. It was the usual early morning ward round on Monday before the start of the full day theatre list. Like always the boss arrived right on time, and with everyone in attention the team walked behind him to see the first patient (Mr S) on the first bed of a twenty-bedded ward.

Mr S – a sixty five-year old man, was due to have anterior resection for rectal cancer (removal of rectum and distal colon and joining the cut end of colon to anal canal). Instead of suturing the cut ends of the bowel by hand, on this occasion the boss was going to use a new gadget known as the staple gun. The company representative had brought the instrument specifically for him to try for the first time.

As we approached the patient's bedside, smilingly he glanced at the patient and at the same time asked me, "Have you arranged with the company representative to bring the gun which we are going to try today?"

"Yes, I have," was my prompt reply.

Without any further conversation with the patient or with anyone else he walked briskly to the next bed and everyone followed. The ward-round finished in about 20 minutes and the whole party left the ward for theatre.

The porter went to the ward to fetch Mr S. However, the nurse phoned theatre to say that Mr S had packed his bags and had gone home, soon after we left the ward. On hearing this I went to investigate.

"Why did he leave?" I asked the ward nurse.

"He had heard on the ward round from you guys that you would be testing a new gun on him. He was terrified that you might shoot some of his vital bits."

"What vital bits?" I asked.

"I don't know – that is what he said. He decided to pack his belongings and left; despite my pleas he refused to stay."

Absence of communication can sometimes end up in a humiliating situation – even for the mighty and the powerful. There is always someone who makes his feelings known.

I PREFER HOME TREATMENT (FROM HA, INDIA, 1992)

During my medical student days it was common practice to have clinical teaching at the bedside of a patient. One would learn to take the clinical history, conduct a physical examination and elicit physical signs. Led by the clinical teacher a large group of students would crowd around the bed with the patient seated in the centre. Most patients didn't appear to mind it – I guess they had no other choice.

I was one of the medical students waiting expectantly on a surgical ward for the arrival of the big boss for a dose of bedside surgical teaching. This was my second term in surgery; I already had a taste of Prof D's grilling teaching techniques during my previous term.

Prof D – six feet tall, bespectacled, broad shouldered giant of a man, arrived on time. Everything in the vicinity of his steps appeared to bow to his presence. A chair had already been stationed close to the bed, where the teaching was due to take place.

The occupant of the bed was a frail old man wearing a lungi (a loose cloth) that covered the lower half of his body. The boss made himself comfortable in the chair and looked all round at the crowd of students over his thick framed glasses. By then we had formed a circle around the bed. Since there were no curtains around any of the beds on the wards those days, the cordon helped to maintain a sense of privacy and dignity. The patient welcomed Prof D with a greeting and a smile and it appeared that they knew each other quite well. He suffered from enlarged prostate and was due to have an operation for that during the next few days.

Prof D began by teaching the prostatic anatomy. Following that, with the patient lying on his left side and with his legs crouched against his chest, one by one he asked us to examine the patient's prostate with a finger placed in his rectum, and describe the findings. Some of us got the findings half right, but most got it wrong, because we could not regurgitate word to word what he had taught us a little while earlier. We had no other option but to bear his verbal onslaught.

During all this time no one thought of the poor old man who had suffered an hour of torture. He was lying quietly on his side in foetal position and appeared to be at peace with himself, until the boss touched him gently and informed him that his services were no longer required.

The graceful old man straightened himself, sat up, adjusted his lungi and gently moved out of his bed. Standing in front of Prof D and looking directly into his eyes, he said, "Sir, I have been here for three days. Yesterday you brought one group of doctors to treat me and today you brought another. If I knew that fingering my backside is the treatment for my bladder condition, I would not have come into the hospital."

The chief was dumbfounded. There was total silence for a couple of minutes, and without a frown on his face the patient collected his belongings and walked out. As he left he still had the decency of wishing everyone good-bye.

Miscommunication is equally problematic. The speaker might think that the right information has been conveyed but the listener may have an entirely different understanding of what was said. Furthermore we tend to forget that patients have no knowledge of technical aspects of surgery and a lack of clear explanation can sometimes lead to confusion and misunderstanding.

During the late seventies I was working at an Iranian hospital. The outpatient department was located in a long rectangular hall that was surrounded by a row of consultation rooms on three sides. During peak morning hours the hall resembled a crowded railway station – full of people, patients and their relatives. The main crowd would assemble around a large central office, which looked very much like a large cage. With deafening noise all round everyone present would try to get the attention of one of the three clerks seated within the enclosure to get a coupon which was the passport that guaranteed a consultation with a doctor on the day. After getting the coupon, the next hurdle was to gain entry into the doctors' consulting rooms. Despite the presence of large and muscular gatekeepers at the entrance door to each room, the fittest, the strongest and the wealthiest managed to push their way into the rooms. The weak and the infirm had to wait.

The penultimate patient to enter my consulting room on the day was a fit but rather frail old man in his mid-seventies who had been referred from about one hundred miles away with acute urinary retention, secondary to a large benign prostate. The referring doctor had already catheterised him and the catheter was connected to a urine bag. Clear urine was draining freely into the bag. His grandson – tall and bubbly, rather smart and well-dressed man in his mid-twenties, accompanied the patient. He answered most of my questions.

After a physical examination I advised the man that he needed prostatectomy (surgical removal of prostate), which is a major surgical undertaking. I concluded by stating that as per the strict hospital rules it was necessary for the family to donate two bottles of blood, since there was a strong possibility of blood loss during surgery for which a blood transfusion might be required. On hearing that the grandson became quite unhappy; he wanted his granddad to be admitted straightaway. However, I insisted that the hospital protocol stipulated that unless arrangements for blood transfusion were made, admission could not take place. "Please arrange two bottles of blood and your granddad will be admitted," I said to him.

Reluctantly the patient and his grandson had to agree. As the grandson was leaving he remarked, "Doctor, I will be back."

A few days later both of them returned. After barging into the consulting room the grandson announced proudly, "Sir, you wanted two bottles of blood, here they are." He proudly got out of his bag two glass-bottles. Each was about three quarters full. In the bottom half of each bottle were decanted blood cells and in the top half was amber coloured plasma. I could not believe my eyes but after recovering from the shock of what was in front of me, I asked the young man, "Where did you get the blood from?"

"Sir, we killed two goats and collected blood in bottles. Sorry, we could not fill the bottles completely because some of it spilled on the floor," he replied apologetically.

I asked the two men to wait, went to the hospital director and narrated the story to him. He advised me to admit the patient and directed the head of pathology to issue blood from the blood bank if it was needed. He also called the grandson to his office and clarified the misunderstanding. The goats' blood was disposed of quietly. Fortunately the surgical procedure was uneventful and the patient did not need any transfusion during or after surgery. After the incident I always made it a point to use the phrase *human blood* in my conversations.

Missing an important word or using a clumsy word, or a poorly phrased, incomplete or inadequately explained sentence, can translate into a funny or an embarrassing episode that may generate a good laugh but can also cause discomfiture at the patient-clinician interface.

THE WRONG SHAVE (FROM DM, NIGERIA, 1988)

I was working as a junior surgical resident at a teaching hospital. A bearded older looking man in his late fifties presented with a large inguinal hernia for which he was offered a date for admission for surgery. A tuft of long, thick and curly hair covered his entire scrotal and pubic areas, and as he was about to leave, the boss said to him, "By the way, can you please shave all the hair two days before the day of your operation?"

The patient returned on the appointed date with a clean-shaven head, neck and face; the pubic and scrotal areas were untouched. The job was eventually undertaken in theatre by the boss himself, which took him as long as the operation itself.

TOO BIG TO SWALLOW (FROM SM, UK, 1990)

A patient complained to me about my registrar – who had seen him on an earlier outpatient visit –, and said, "Your understudy was not thinking when he prescribed me the tablets. They are too big to swallow. Therefore I cut them into two halves with a kitchen knife, and only then I was able to consume them." On enquiry it emerged that the medication under discussion was actually a glycerine suppository.

THE WIND DIRECTION (FROM TC, SCOTLAND, 1999)

This was my first job as a house officer. Led by the chief, the team arrived at the bedside of a man in his seventies, who had undergone an operation for bowel perforation two days before. After the usual greetings the chief asked the patient, "Did you pass wind?"

After a rotational movement of his head with his nostrils wide open the gentleman replied, "Come to think of it I can actually smell it, but it was certainly not me; it must be one of you."

YOU SCREAM – I SCREAM (FROM ZF, UK, 2004)

I was working as a staff grade urologist and was performing video-urodynamic investigation on a cheerful lady in her mid-forties. The procedure is done without any general or regional anaesthesia and involves catheterising the patient's bladder and filling it through the catheter with fluid diluted with radio-opaque contrast. As the bladder is filled, changes in bladder pressure are recorded and at the same time the bladder is screened (and x-rayed if necessary) to check for any structural abnormalities. During the procedure the person performing the test communicates regularly with the patient and the radiographer.

After filling the patient's bladder with contrast fluid I said to the radiographer, "Screen please." Instantly the patient screamed at the top of her voice. Not only was everyone taken aback but in the process the urinary catheter slipped out of her bladder.

"Why did you do that?" I asked.

"You asked me to scream and I screamed," she said in a fit of laughter.

After everyone else had a laugh we started all over again.

It is sometimes difficult to decide how technical one needs to be when explaining a disease process, an operative procedure or a treatment plan. Oversimplifying technical jargon can lead to confusion, and talking in riddles can make matters equally complicated.

Mr S – a carpenter in his mid-fifties attended my clinic for a follow-up consultation. I had operated on him for radical cystectomy (removal of urinary bladder) and orthotopic bladder substitution (reconstructing a new bladder from the patient's own bowel) for treatment of bladder cancer a few weeks before. The post-operative period had been uneventful; the wound had healed nicely and the pathology report of the excised specimen was favourable. The family was pleased with the way things had gone. From my point of view one of the important questions to ask was how the new bladder was functioning?

"I am getting there slowly, I can generate a urinary flow and can empty my new bladder by applying pressure on my tummy. I am quite happy Mr M." "As you said to me before the operation the new bladder is made from my bowel, which is a totally different material than a normal bladder and may not function as effectively as the natural bladder."

After a pause he added, "If I remember correctly you said it is like asking a 'mason to do a carpenter's job'. You did say that, didn't you?"

"Yes I did," I replied.

Following that we carried on with the rest of the consultation – discussed future follow-up arrangements, the histology result, nutritional needs and bladder training. As he was leaving the room he turned back, walked a couple of steps towards me and said, "Mr M, do you know that I am a carpenter by trade?"

"I know that Mr S."

"I hope you don't mind me saying this: A mason can never do a carpenter's job. Therefore comparing the new bladder to a mason is not correct," he said with conviction.

"Umm... I guess you are right..." I mumbled.

"I have been in the carpentry trade for forty five years and would like to reiterate that a mason can never do a carpenter's job. I hope you don't mind me saying, I don't think you should use that phrase when you explain the operation to your future patients, and I mean that."

I tried to conclude the consultation by saying, "Thank you so much Mr S for pointing that out." However, he carried on, "Mr M, can I also suggest that instead of saying 'a mason doing a carpenter's job' you should say 'a handyman doing a carpenter's job'. I have been thinking about this; you see a handyman can do some carpentry but a mason can't. You know what I mean."

"Thank you for your suggestion, I appreciate it," I replied.

After that day I never used the phrase again.

A somewhat similar incident happened on another occasion a few years before. Mr K, a recently retired electrical contractor in his mid-sixties, was under my care for many years. I had operated on him for nephro-ureterectomy (removal of kidney and the entire tube connecting the kidney to urinary bladder) for cancer arising from the lining of the kidney tubes. We came to know each other quite well over the years.

Mr K developed similar tumours in the bladder, which were removed with the use of an endoscope through the urethra (water passage), without an open operation. In order to prevent future regrowth of such tumours it was decided to treat him with instillations of a drug into the bladder at weekly intervals. I explained the plan of action to him during the outpatient consultation. "Mr K, there is a risk that these tumours might come back and in order to reduce the risk of recurrence it is necessary that at weekly intervals we instil the drug in liquid form into your bladder through a catheter."

"How long does the drug stay in the bladder and how does it work?" he asked.

"You will have to try to retain the drug in the bladder for a couple of hours so that it acts on the bladder lining. Like a weed killer that does not allow weeds to regrow in the garden, the drug reduces the risk of these tumours growing again."

The first two instillations were uneventful but after the third instillation he became quite ill and developed severe bladder symptoms – painful urgency and frequency of micturition.

"That bloody weed killer of yours killed me – almost!" he said when he came to see me.

"Sorry, Mr K, the drug can sometimes cause bladder inflammation what is known as chemical cystitis, that is a well-known complication of this treatment. I did warn you about that," I said defensively.

"I don't care what you said, but that weed killer of yours is poisonous stuff. Well, a weed killer is a poison, isn't it?" he said angrily.

"It is not a weed killer Mr K," I tried to plead.

I tried my best to explain but the outcome of the meeting

was unsatisfactory. Thankfully his symptoms improved over the next few days, and after a few subsequent clinical encounters we became friendly again. But on each visit he used to remind me subtly how ill he had been after I prescribed the 'weed killer'. I could not convince him that it was a drug and not a weed killer. Needless to add that after that episode I did not use the phrase again.

Improper words, and off the cuff remarks – even the ones that are uttered jokingly, can be construed as serious statements and can hurt feelings. A junior working in Department of Obstetrics in Australia was perplexed when an expectant mother started crying after he informed her that the baby was still in breach position. On enquiry the mother stated that with her husband's help, for the last four weeks she had stood on her head everyday – for half an hour in the morning and half an hour in the evening. On questioning it emerged that at the previous antenatal consultation she had asked the chief if anything could be done to shift the baby from breach position. Apparently, the chief had said (jokingly?), " I don't think so – apart from standing on your head!"

In 1992 a young doctor who had already embarked on a surgical career joined my unit to fill a locum post for a few weeks. He had good references and a great resume – publications in medical journals and, distinctions and prizes at the medical school. He was intelligent, well read and possessed an inquisitive mind, and was a budding academic in the true sense. Yet he shuddered when holding a surgical instrument in theatre and in a very short time it also became clear that he could not handle the most important person – the patient.

When asked by a patient of mine – who was due to be transferred to another hospital to have radiotherapy for treatment of bladder cancer – about what to expect, allegedly he said, "They will fry your bladder in order to kill the cancer within it, Mr J." Crying his heart out, Mr J ran to see the ward sister. Being an old fashioned disciplinarian, after consoling the gentleman she gave the doctor a piece of her mind along with a tutorial on how to talk to patients.

Another day he tried to consent a patient for the procedure of cystolithilopaxy (breaking a stone in the urinary bladder and washing out the fragments through the water passage without the need to cut through the abdomen). Apparently he had said, "We are going to use special equipment to blast to bits the damn thing lying in your bladder!" The patient signed the consent form but refused to accompany the porter to theatre until I went to the ward to talk to him. When I saw him, he was in tears and in a state of panic. He thought there was going to be a loud explosion in his bladder, which would not only shake him but also the whole hospital. After I calmed him down I took the young doctor to one side and had a chat with him.

The junior was clearly tactless as well as insensitive with the usage of his words. Such individuals need to be identified and counselled during their training days lest they grow into unsympathetic adults.

BOOK CHOICE (FROM PT, UK, 1996)

The incident happened during my junior surgical training. The man on bed eight was in his mid-seventies and was diagnosed with advanced pelvic malignancy. Apart from symptomatic control and some palliative radiotherapy no further treatment was being planned. The registrar had broken the bad news to the patient and his wife the night before, but they were keen to speak to the consultant Mr B. This was arranged and at the appointed time Mr B arrived to see them. The wife was sitting by her husband's bedside but both appeared overwhelmed and nervous.

Dressed in a perfectly fitting blue suit with a yellow tie and standing stiffly on the left side of the bed, without any pleasantries whatsoever, Mr B started the conversation by saying,

"I was told by my registrar who spoke to you both yesterday that you wish to speak to me. What do you want to know?"

"Mr B, I have a few questions but there is one question that bothers me most," and after that remark he paused, held his wife's hand tight, and after some hesitation asked nervously, "How long have I got?"

Mr B replied, "Not long, but tell me do you like books?"

"Yes, I do," he replied in a boastful manner.

After a pause Mr B replied, "Well, in that case if you like a good book, I would advise you not to buy Tolstoy's 'War and Peace' – instead go for a small book – perhaps a small collection of short stories."

There was complete silence on both sides as the patient looked at his wife. And whilst he continued looking and holding her hand tighter, without saying any more Mr B left the ward. The patient and his wife hugged each other as tears rolled down their faces.

That must have been an awful experience for the couple. For the registrar that would have been a lesson about what not to say when breaking bad news. I narrated the anecdote to a cluster of surgeon friends, which opened an interesting debate. While all present agreed that his attitude was uncaring and arrogant, a couple of them felt that comparing life with a book wasn't totally out of order. They also thought that the news had to be conveyed openly and in a straight manner. The discussion then moved on to situations when a clinician needs to spell out the truth and at the same time be assertive. Out of the few stories that were given as examples the following one stood out.

THE BRAINTEASER (FROM GF, UK, 2007)

I was working as a junior registrar for Mr C – a very well respected vascular surgeon. One day he asked me to see a patient in the clinic – a pleasant lady in her early sixties who looked much older than her years. Her elderly husband accompanied her. She had suffered left sided stroke in the past and had been experiencing further episodes of transient giddiness. A duplex ultrasound scan had demonstrated critical blockage in the left common carotid artery (a large blood vessel in the neck that supplies blood to the brain), and it was clear that the blood vessel required unblocking – a procedure known as carotid endarterectomy. After examining her I explained that she would require an operation to reduce the risk of a further stroke.

"Oh no, doctor. I don't want any operation; thank you very much. Never had one in mee life – and never intend on 'avin one. If the good Lord sees it fit to end mee life then so be it," she responded with a broad grin of disapproval on her face.

I tried to rationalise with her and explained that the operation would allow her to preserve what independence she currently had. However she wasn't budging. I then tried to make her understand that a further stroke could make her even more dependent on her elderly husband, who was listening thoughtfully to the conversation. At that point he intervened and tried to persuade her but she was steadfast in her resolve of not having any kind of surgery. "I would rather bee dead!" She said categorically.

Dejected I went to explain the situation to Mr C who listened to me attentively but didn't say a word. When I finished speaking he stood up abruptly and walked out of the room. I followed him to where the lady was sitting in a chair. He looked at her husband and shook his hand and then turned to the patient and said, "Madam, you have already lost half of your brain. I know that you are a very intelligent woman but even you need half a brain to function." After a measured pause and with a smile he added, "And therefore I won't take no for an answer from you. Is that understood?" He was measured and firm but not rude.

The lady's husband burst out laughing, and then Mrs X started laughing. To my utter amazement, she acquiesced and after shaking her hand Mr C walked out without saying a further word. For the apprentice (me) this was a tutorial on assertiveness that was delivered on the shop floor.

The junior must have thought what the boss differently that made the lady agree to have the procedure? He wasn't rude or loud but he was firm and convincing and the message was delivered in a clear and calculated manner. The language, the tone of speech and words combined to make it effective and well received. Whilst he was self-assured, the patient's interest was his first priority. The incident demonstrated assertiveness, which is goal driven behaviour; the 'book choice' episode described earlier typified arrogance – that is a manifestation of emotionally driven behaviour.

These days surgeons and surgical trainees move from one country to another to seek better career or training opportunities and in some cases it becomes necessary for them to learn a new language in a new country. In some countries the regulatory body (like the General Medical Council in the UK), tests the language competency of a foreign doctor rigorously. Even if you are already fluent in the native language of the adopted country it still takes time for the doctor to grasp common expressions and colloquial phrases. For instance it takes a while for an immigrant to the UK to realise that stomach and abdomen can mean the same thing, and so can heart and ticker, that pain in nuts, balls, nuggets, goolies, cobblers or marbles denotes pain in the testes, and blood in pee or water signifies blood in urine. It also takes the newcomer time to realise that people in different towns and cities speak in different accents and dialects, which can sometimes lead to difficulties.

A WEE BIT (FROM GD, SCOTLAND, 1996)

With a big bundle of hospital notes in his hands a young immigrant Asian doctor who had started his first senior house officer job interrupted me politely in a busy outpatient clinic.

"Sir, the patient in my room says that his name is V B Ruff, but the name on the notes is different. When I asked the receptionist she says there is no Mr Ruff on the clinic list."

I walked to the doctor's room where I found a middle-aged man lying on a couch and gazing vacantly at the ceiling with his left hand holding his head. He looked quite unwell.

"Mr D, what did you tell the young doctor your name was?" I asked the patient.

"He did not ask me my name. I think he asked me how I was," he replied shakily.

"Okay my friend, what did you answer?"

"Wee – bee – rough. That is all, I said."

I examined the patient and arranged his admission to the hospital, and after his exit from the room said to the doctor, "Don't take it to heart, young man. Scottish accent can sometimes be difficult to understand – even for people born and brought up in England."

Occasionally the immigrant is confronted by cultural dilemmas. A UK surgeon remembered asking his junior trainee from Middle Eastern origin for a clinical report regarding a patient on whom he had undertaken prostatectomy. Struggling with his words the junior replied, "Not very good sir, drop, drop, drop – like tip, tip, tip…" And he demonstrated the falling drops with rhythmic movements of his right index finger. When the boss advised him that the English word for 'tip-tip-tip' was a 'dribble', he replied, "I know that sir but I can't say that – that would be utterly disrespectful, because the patient's name is Mr Dribble."

Another surgical colleague was not keen to extend the tenure of his senior house officer who was born and qualified from Nigeria. The reason was that he thought the doctor was very shy and unfriendly. When asked how he came to that conclusion, he replied that the doctor never looked him in the eye. However, he changed his mind when his anaesthetic colleague of West African roots told him that people from that part of the world tend not to gaze directly at their superiors because that is perceived as confrontational and rude.

It is not only the communication between the staff and patients, and their loved ones that matters but also the exchange amongst the staff on the front line. A healthcare facility such as a hospital is the hub of a vast communication network that receives, processes, relays and responds to large numbers of queries, messages and other chunks of information from numerous sources every day. Sometimes a piece of information has to traverse across a number of intermediary nexuses before reaching its final destination. Incongruence at any point along the line can create turbulence or even an explosion in the whole circuit. I learnt that lesson many years ago.

Just after finishing a case in the operating theatre I was handed a note that had been left by one of my enthusiastic senior house officers which read: "Mr M, Mrs T is in a state – the family are all by her bedside and they are literally up in arms. They wish to speak to you urgently." I had undertaken a reconstructive bladder procedure on Mrs T a couple of weeks earlier that involved making her bladder larger by patching it with an isolated segment of bowel – the operation known as enterocystoplasty. The procedure involves suturing of the bowel edges to those of the bisected bladder.

The surgical operation had been uneventful and there were no post-operative complications. She was discharged home with a catheter draining urine from the bladder, and was to be readmitted a few days later to have a bladder X-ray (cystogram). That involves filling the bladder with contrast fluid and checking whether the suture line (join) has healed completely, so that the catheter can be removed. Mrs T had been readmitted on this day for cystography and provided the X-ray was okay the catheter would be removed.

In view of the urgency of the message I went to see the patient on the ward on my own – the senior house officer was busy with another patient on another ward. However, before going into the side room where Mrs T was admitted, the ward sister stopped me and warned that even though the patient was clinically fine she and her family were very anxious and upset. At that point I didn't quite know why that was so.

The ward sister and I went into the room together where I found Mrs T lying comfortably in bed. On seeing me tears started flowing down her eyes. Her husband – who was standing nearby, was quiet and appeared to be full to the brim with pent-up anger. The body language of the extended family gathered around her bed was also intimidating; the whole atmosphere was extraordinarily tense.

"Good afternoon Mrs T, how are you doing?" I asked.

"How did that happen?" she replied in anguish.

Before I could answer, the husband interjected, " Yes, we need explanations. How did my wife's bladder rupture?" Soon after, the family joined in a chorus with everyone demanding answers from me.

Feeling rather overwhelmed and almost speechless, and not knowing what had happened, I somehow managed to persuade the relatives to stay outside the room until I examined Mrs T. The ward sister remained in the room with me.

Mrs T had no symptoms or signs of bladder rupture – she was not in pain, the abdomen was soft, flat and non-tender and the abdominal wound had healed nicely. I could not understand the reason for the unhappiness and asked, "Mrs T, who told you that your bladder is ruptured?"

"Your understudy," she replied sharply.

"Let me assure you that you do not have a bladder rupture. You are fine. I will have a look at the X-ray and then decide when the catheter should be taken out," I said reassuringly.

After I walked out of the room, I met the family. After a difficult time initially I was able to calm them down too. Thereafter I went straight to the imaging department where I found the radiologist who had performed the X-ray. He and I had a look at the X-ray together. It showed a tiny, pinhead size leak of contrast from a single point along the bladder suture line.

Returning to the ward I explained to the patient and the family the true state of affairs with the aid of a diagram drawn on a sheet of paper – showing the bladder with the patch of bowel sutured to it and the pinhead sized leak. I advised her to go home and come back for removal of catheter in a couple of days. Two days later the catheter was removed and she passed urine without any problems. Her presenting symptoms for which she had the operation had improved markedly. She and her family remained grateful for the care that she had received for many years thereafter.

I decided to investigate the incident to unearth the sequence of events that had led to confusion.

During the x-ray procedure the radiologist had apparently commented to the radiographer that there was a "tiny leak" of contrast at one point along the suture line. The radiographer apparently ignored the adjective and conveyed to the nurse who came to collect the patient that there was a "'leak from the bladder". The nurse changed the noun and communicated to her colleagues on the ward during the handover that there was a "hole in the bladder". The news percolated to everyone on the ward, and the senior house officer on duty was contacted by one of the other nurses with the news that the x-ray had shown that Mrs T's "'bladder was ruptured'".

Without examining the patient the senior house officer put up an intravenous drip and advised Mrs T to rest in bed, stop eating and drinking. She also told her that the x-ray had shown evidence of "bladder rupture." On hearing these words Mrs T was naturally terrified, so she rang her husband at work. After a few more phone calls the alarming news was transmitted to the whole family who descended on the ward in large numbers.

Oral communication is spontaneous and has a short thinking

time, and spoken words are like bullets – once released from the barrel they cannot be retrieved. In contrast, written communication offers the sender the opportunity to pause, to reflect and to choose words carefully before transmitting the information to the receiver. It entails appropriate selection and arrangement of words and phrases, and cohesive composition of sentences. As a general rule written communication is more valid and reliable than speech; it is also a permanent means of exchange that provides ready records and references. Good defence in medical negligence claims or Fitness to Practise Tribunal hearings hinges upon a good written record that is factual, rational and legible.

In the West a large volume of written correspondence passes from the primary to secondary care and vice versa, and mistakes at the points of interaction between the two are not uncommon, usually in the form of a missed letter, an erroneous word or a misguided phrase. Such errors can arise in both strands of care.

A general practitioner wrote to a urologist: "Mr X was under your car [sic: care] last year and since then he has developed a penile condition, please see and advise." The urologist wrote back: "Thanks for your referral regarding Mr X who needs circumcision for Balanitis Erotica Obliterans [sic: Xerotica]."

Silly errors can sometimes spiral into further exchanges and even generate a debate, as in the following incident from my own practice.

Mr B was under my care for many years for cancer of prostate. He was managed with the usual combination of treatments: surgery, radiation and medication – hormones and chemotherapy. The tumour had spread to his liver and bones and all options of active treatment had been exhausted. I explained the poor prognosis to the patient and his wife. We also discussed the need for supportive care in the primary care setting. I concluded by saying to the couple that there was no need for further hospital appointments. The news did not come as a surprise to them.

After their departure I dictated a letter to Mr B's GP, whose first name was Christopher. The letter that was typed and posted by my secretary without anyone else checking, read as follows:

Dear Christ [sic: Chris]

> *I saw Mr B today. Unfortunately the disease is now too advanced... There is little that I can offer, and therefore I have not made any further arrangements for his follow-up with me... I am discharging him back to your kind care.*

I did not know about the typing error in the letter until the GP phoned me two days later to seek clarification. When I realised the mistake I started apologising. However, he responded by saying, "Please don't be sorry; I understand that it was a typing error, but I feel that Mr B's transfer of care suggested by you is quite appropriate. As a matter of fact I showed your letter to Mr B and he feels exactly the same."

When I narrated the details of our conversation to my secretary, she was upset at herself and rang Mr B to apologise. However, Mr B could not understand why she was apologising.

As in most professions medics invent their own set of acronyms that they use for correspondence, some of which can be quite confusing, particularly for newcomers. For instance some surgical bosses are best known by their acronyms. Phrases like *admit under GRM, to be discussed with GRM,* are commonly recorded in hospital notes. Such acronyms are easy to decipher, but over the years the use of acronyms has multiplied which can make life difficult, especially for senior members of the tribe. Here is a page from an actual hospital record:

SR-74
HOPI: C/o – – SOB
H/O – – – – TURP (BPH) 2/52

TEDS+
H/O - - - HTN
PMH- - - RIH, TKR- - R
E?? . LBBB, LVH
Urine A, U&E, FBC, KUB, CXR, LFT:- WNL
PD:- PE/MI/CAP
D/W Reg:- Arrange CS, start AB - - (Aug IV)
signed
786

The decrypted version is as follows:

SR (patient's name) 74 years old

History of present illness: complains of shortness of breath

History of transurethral resection of prostate for benign prostatic hyperplasia two weeks before

Thrombo-embolic deterrent stockings are on

History of hypertension

Past medical history of right inguinal hernia and total knee replacement, right side

Electrocardiogram shows left bundle branch block and left ventricular hypertrophy

Urine analysis, urea and electrolytes, full blood count, kidney-ureter-bladder (abdominal X-ray), chest X-ray, liver function tests: within normal limits

Provisional diagnosis: pulmonary embolism/myocardial infarction/community acquired pneumonia

Discussed with registrar who advised to arrange clotting screen and to start on antibiotics (Augmentin intravenous)

Signature

Bleep Number 786

Each country has its own acronymic language that the immigrant doctor has to learn after arrival in the adopted land. For example: BMF (basic metabolic profile) in the US is U&E (urea &

electrolytes) in the UK; CBC (comprehensive blood count) in the US is FBC (full blood count) in the UK; NO (nil orally) in the US is NBM (nil by mouth) in the UK, and so on.

Confusion is also compounded when one abbreviation represents two different expressions. For instance: PID is prolapsed intervertebral disc and Pelvic Inflammatory Disease; TLC is Tender Loving Care and Total Leucocyte (white blood cell) Count; DOA is Date Of Admission and Dead On Arrival; RIP is Raised Intracranial Pressure as well as Rest In Peace; and there are many more. The problem is that new acronyms are invented all the time and a clinician has to keep up with the rapidly expanding acronymic vocabulary. Because of rising number of medico-legal and Fitness To Practise (FTP) cases, in the future lawyers, tribunalists and managers dealing with medical mishaps and claims will have to be well versed with the acronymic language of medicine.

Some written errors are the cause of embarrassment, and some a source of humorous pastime for everyone. However, a small typing mistake like *didn't* instead of *did*, or *without* instead of *with* can lead to potentially disastrous consequences. The likelihood of such mistakes is greater with the use of voice recognition and remote typing pools but the policy of copying the correspondence to patients, which enhances the prospects of the letter being checked carefully before being sent, should help to reduce the incidence of such errors.

Misreading is more common with handwritten exchanges and doctors are well known for illegible handwriting. Some would argue that poor handwriting is because of time constraints, as doctors have to record in detail each clinical encounter in a short space of time. However, illegible writing is a significant cause of hazard in medical and surgical care and an important patient safety issue. There are numerous examples of this in the medico-legal literature. In the following case recounted by a colleague an agile pair of eyes averted a disaster – just in time!

A MEATY KIDNEY (FROM NG, INDIA, 2005)

This was during my residency – the early days of laparoscopic (keyhole) surgery. A fifty year-old lady was admitted under care of Dr B – recently appointed, young and enthusiastic consultant surgeon. The patient complained of recurrent left loin pain for a few years. The handwritten ultrasound report stated that the patient had a small contracted left kidney, and the renogram (isotope kidney scan) report read: "no functioning kidney tissue seen on the left side." It was therefore concluded that she had a left small contracted non-functioning kidney. Arrangements were made for patient's admission for left nephrectomy (kidney removal) by keyhole surgery.

After positioning and placing of the ports and the camera the left kidney was exposed. While the surgeon was dissecting around the kidney, naively a medical student who was present in theatre asked Dr G, "Sir, the ultrasound report suggests a 'small contracted left kidney', why does the exposed kidney appear quite meaty and of normal size?" After a sharp glance at the student Dr G paused and looked at the ultrasound report and appeared to agree with the student's observation by saying, "You are damn right!"

Dr B checked the handwritten ultrasound report again. The actual wording on the report was: "Normal lt [sic: left] kidney. There may be a small contracted rt [sic: right] kidney." However, the writing was so illegible that the words lt and rt could be easily mistaken for each other. Erroneously the senior resident wrote in the notes as well as the renogram request form, "Patient complains of pain in left kidney area. Ultrasound shows possibly a small contracted lt [instead of rt] kidney."

The mistake in the handwritten ultrasound report was carried forward unabated in every subsequent clinical record. The chain of errors was realised just in time and the only functioning normal left kidney saved – courtesy of the watchful student.

The above example echoes the sad incident in similar circumstances at a Welsh hospital referred to earlier. In that instance the error was apparently transferred from a hospital admittance slip and carried on to the operating theatre list, eventually ending with a disastrous outcome – with the patient losing the good kidney instead of the cancerous one.

The moral is that good communication is the passport to the practice of safe surgery. It is a two-stage process: that is receiving and responding. A good communicator is a good listener who has the ability to dissect the information package carefully, separate fact from fiction and communicate back decisions as well as feelings with compassion and care. Effective oral communication also means conveying negative or difficult messages without creating a conflict or a barrier, and without dismantling mutual trust. It is also essential that the clinician's body language does not negate the message – kind and sympathetic words spoken without emotion mean nothing to the listener.

Present day surgeons are fully aware that patients need to be treated as individuals and not as numbers, and that they must be fully informed and supported in order that they can make meaningful decisions and choices about their treatment and care. There are now courses and seminars available on the subject for all healthcare workers but ultimately it all boils down to common sense, which is much more than simply talking to patients about their diagnosis and potential treatments but to look at the world through their eyes. From my experience as a healthcare manager I firmly believe that bad or ineffective communication or lack of communication are the root causes of a large proportion of complaints in healthcare. Notwithstanding the efforts of healthcare strategists and communication experts, mistakes due to poor communication continue to happen in the surgical world. This is an area about which clinicians, including surgeons, are sometimes casual and therefore vulnerable.

In due course electronic clinical records will probably make doctors' handwriting and scribbled records an out-dated exercise. Paperless records held on computers and hand held devices have already been adopted by many hospitals in the West. But are we on a safer footing with these newer tools? Inadvertent typing errors coupled with impulsive transmission of records can compromise patient safety and data confidentiality. The exciting new world of information technology is unquestionably smarter but it is certainly not securer. A serious untoward incident is only a click or a ping away!

11

MYSTERIES, MIRACLES & MYTHS

This was late morning on a Saturday during the late 1990s. After having finished the procedure of radical prostatectomy (removal of prostate for cancer) on Mr T, I made myself comfortable in a chair in the theatre recovery area with a cup of tea, and was about to start writing the operation notes. The operation had gone very well with no intra-operative complications. However, as soon as I started putting pen to paper I was informed by one of the recovery nurses that during Mr T's transfer from the operating table to a trolley the urinary catheter balloon had deflated spontaneously resulting in the catheter slipping out from his bladder. I rushed back to theatre and found the patient on a theatre trolley with the anaesthetist standing at the head end. He was breathing normally but was still unconscious and had not recovered fully from the effect of general anaesthetic.

Using lubricating jelly impregnated with a local anaesthetic for the urethra (water passage), I reinserted a new catheter into his bladder without any difficulty. However, as I was connecting the catheter to a urine bag, suddenly the patient stopped breathing and turned blue. My anaesthetic colleague promptly reinserted a tube into his windpipe, connected it to an anaesthetic machine and started pumping oxygen into his lungs. We nursed Mr T in theatre recovery area hoping that he would start breathing spontaneously soon, which would allow the breathing tube to be removed. However, that didn't happen and by early evening the situation worsened; his pupils became fully dilated and unresponsive and he remained completely impassive to any external stimuli. I informed Mr T's wife and daughter about the state of affairs and we decided to shift him to the intensive care unit (ICU) for respiratory and other organ support.

Mr T remained in deep coma with no change in his physical state or neurological status over the next four days. With each day I got increasingly anxious about him. Of particular concern to me and to my other clinical colleagues were his fixed dilated pupils. A case conference was held involving urology, neurology and intensive care teams. Following that we had a meeting with his wife and daughter at which I raised concerns regarding Mr T's chances of recovery. The family were distressed which was understandable. However, they didn't know how stressed I was about the situation – I had to put up a bold exterior.

I visited Mr T in the ICU twice a day everyday, first thing in the morning and before I left the hospital in the evening. On my evening visit on the fifth post-operative day there was no change in his clinical state and in my mind I was becoming despondent about his chances of recovery.

On the sixth post-operative morning as I arrived on the ICU for my routine visit, I heard a lot of commotion near Mr T's bed. As I made my way through a ring of people standing around his bed I was shocked to see Mr T half reclined in his bed shouting and swearing angrily at the top of his voice. On seeing me he yelled, "I am glad you are here Mr M, I want my b... breakfast. I am f... hungry, but these f... people are refusing to give it to me; I need to know why!"

"Okay, what would you like to have for your breakfast Mr T?" I tried to calm him down.

"What I always have – cereal with milk and toast," he shouted back.

"Okay, we will order cereal with milk and toast for you, Mr T."

Whilst waiting for breakfast to arrive, the night nurse informed me that at about six o'clock that morning Mr T had woken up suddenly. He had pulled the breathing tube and after a few coughs had started talking and demanding breakfast.

I continued my conversation with Mr T – about him and his family. He seemed to answer all my questions correctly until I asked him, "And by the way, what day is it today Mr T?" Promptly he replied, "It is Saturday, of course!" The days during which he had been comatose had passed him by.

By now breakfast arrived and as he started eating and I left the unit feeling totally relieved and elated.

He was moved to the main ward where I visited him again in the evening. This time he was much calmer, back to his normal self. His family had already visited him and he had been informed about what had happened. I told Mr T how delighted I had been to see him fight for his breakfast earlier that day, even though my words couldn't describe fully the enormity of my joy. He told me how happy he was to come back, realising that he had lost a few days of his life. I was about to say, "Mr T, perhaps I also lost a few days of my life." However, I decided to keep quiet. After a couple of days he was discharged home in a fit state – a happy ending to a suspenseful story.

Mr T remained cancer free for many years thereafter and came to see me for follow-up twice every year. I always greeted him with the sentence, "What day is it today Mr T?" And he always replied, "It is Saturday, of course!"

How did that happen? What led to a sudden change in Mr T's *Milieu Intérieur* that woke him up suddenly? I kept thinking about the episode for many days thereafter but could not answer the question. We discussed the case in our clinical meeting where colleagues came up with various hypotheses, but no one had a proper scientific explanation. It remains a mystery for me even today. Was that a miracle or simply a state of ignorance about a scientific explanation?

A miracle is described as a beneficial phenomenon that cannot be clearly explained by known laws of nature. A medical miracle refers to a remarkable event that is unanticipated and inexplicable, which occurs against all odds, despite being outside the range of known medical or scientific expectations. Regardless of one's belief in miracles and supernatural powers, in a surgeon's world, clinical events for which there is no clear explanation do happen from time to time. These may simply represent a lack of understanding but such incidents do make a clinician pause, reflect and wonder. Here are a few more examples from other sources.

HOW WAS THE PARTY? (FROM RK, INDIA, 1982)

A vibrant young man in his forties was admitted for investigation and treatment of a complex problem related to his bowels. Soon he became friendly with all junior doctors of which I was one. At that time three enthusiastic medical students were attached to our firm. All trainees and bosses liked them and taught them regularly. This was the last week of their clinical attachment with us.

After investigations it was decided that the patient needed complex bowel surgery, which was undertaken under general anaesthetic. The students watched the surgical procedure with interest. During the latter part of the operation whilst the patient was still under general anaesthetic and everyone present was in a relaxed mood, they expressed the wish to go for an evening meal with the surgical team. Everyone agreed with the suggestion and a discussion about the choice of the restaurant followed.

A couple of days later during the ward round, out of the blue the patient asked, "How was the party?" and whilst we looked at one another he came out with a supplementary, "And how was the food at the restaurant of your choice?"

We initially thought that he was hallucinating. However, on further questioning he told us about the various restaurant options that we had discussed, and how we agreed about the final choice of the venue. It was clear that he had listened to the entire conversation that took place whilst we were working on him in theatre when he was deeply anaesthetised. We felt very uncomfortable.

Perhaps noticing our unease he added hastily, "It was odd. I could hear everything but couldn't do anything. Mind you, I enjoyed it and wanted to join in the conversation. And, trust me, I was not in pain or discomfort at all."

That was reassuring for all of us.

KEEP SMILING (FROM HG, POLAND, 2000)

The extraordinary incident happened at a teaching hospital where I used to work as a junior anaesthetist. A comatose male patient in his thirties, who had been involved in a serious road traffic accident and had suffered brain stem injury, was admitted to a two-bedded bay in the ICU. The other bed was empty.

The patient remained in coma on a ventilator for many weeks and developed multi-organ failure. On this particular day it was decided on the morning ward round to get the patient reassessed by the neurology team. After a thorough examination they pronounced him brain-dead and discussions were held with the family regarding withdrawal of ventilatory and other organ support.

During the late afternoon on the same day, due to non-availability of beds in the hospital a lady in her mid-twenties had to be admitted to the other empty bed in the same bay. She was in a comatose state due to alcohol and drug overdose. By early evening she started recovering but was still disorientated.

The nurse who was looking after both patients left the bay unattended for a few minutes and on her return she raised an alarm. The delirious young lady had moved from her bed and was lying on top of the comatose man. To everyone's amazement the young man had a big smile on his face and he was also sexually aroused with a full-blown erection. Interestingly soon after the lady was separated from the patient, the smile and sexual arousal disappeared and his face became rigid again. Even though respiratory and other organ support was continued, sadly the young man died during the early hours of next morning.

THE FOUR Ps (IK, PAKISTAN, 1976)

This bizarre incident took place more than forty years ago well before the era of sophisticated scan technology. A village girl in her early teens – pretty and innocent looking, and accompanied by her old looking father, was admitted with a short history of loss of weight and appetite, and a distended abdomen secondary to ascites (fluid accumulation in the abdominal cavity). She was the only surviving child and had been brought up by her father because her mother had died a few months after her birth. Abdominal palpation revealed a number of nodular lumps.

It was decided to undertake a laparotomy (surgical exploration of abdomen) and after opening the abdomen many litres of fluid were drained. There were numerous hard nodules present all over the peritoneal cavity, bowel wall and mesentery. Three large pieces were excised for biopsy and the abdomen was closed. The histology result was reported as "lymphosarcoma of intestine".

Literature search revealed this to be a rare but highly malignant tumour with a very poor prognosis. After obtaining a second opinion about the histological diagnosis from another centre of repute, two weeks after the surgical procedure her father was informed about the sad news. He took the news well and accepted it as the "Will of God".

About three months later the old man along with his daughter reappeared in the out-patient department. This time he himself needed help for a large inguinal hernia, which was getting painful intermittently. He had brought his daughter along, partly to look after him during the hospital stay (which is not uncommon in the Asian setting), and partly because there was no one to look after her at home.

Soon after arrangements were made for his admission to the hospital for surgical treatment, attention focused on the young girl who appeared healthy and well. Her abdominal wound had healed, the scar appeared sound and supple, she had gained weight, the abdominal distension had gone and there were no nodules palpable on abdominal examination. Everyone was amazed to see that she was a picture of health. On questioning the father narrated the sequence of events as follows:

"After leaving the hospital we went straight to our village. I took her to my local pir (a Muslim religious figure). He blessed her with prayers and gave her a powder to take, with the instruction to consume about half a teaspoonful of that per day with goat's milk for two weeks. The abdominal swelling started disappearing after one week … and four weeks later everything was back to normal."

Which of the four Ps was responsible for her cure? Was it the magical powder that apparently worked and if so what was in it? Was it the pir's supernatural touch? Or was it his prayer that worked? Or did the pathologists from two different institutions get it wrong? Whatever the explanation the old man had an unshakeable belief that it was the prayer that had saved his daughter's life.

Clinicians are accustomed to hearing from patients and their families statements such as: 'It was touch and go doctor, perhaps it was written in my fate to survive' – 'It was lucky that my wife insisted that I have a blood test' – 'my doctor was brilliant, he got me to see you within a week, that was fortunate!' Such pronouncements are commonly made in situations where the end result of treatment is satisfactory.

Conversely you hear statements like: 'They struggled all night in theatre but couldn't save my wife, they couldn't fight destiny,' – 'It was unlucky that we wasted a few weeks' – 'Unfortunately I suffered from a bad infection' and so on. Such assertions are often heard in circumstances where the outcome of an illness is unfavourable. In both situations, however, the emphasis is on words like fate, destiny, luck and fortune. Good treatment result is attributed to being lucky and bad outcome is believed to be a consequence of misfortune. The carers or clinicians are seen as the facilitators of the individual's preordained plan. Does destiny really matter or is it too simplistic an excuse or explanation for a favourable or an adverse clinical outcome – in other words a coincidence? I have pondered over this question on numerous occasions – in good times as well as in bad.

Many years ago I performed a long and complex abdomino-pelvic surgical operation for bladder cancer on Mr D – a 66 year old fit man. The procedure included removal of urinary bladder with reconstruction of a new bladder from the bowel. The operation involves forming several joins involving the bowel and the urinary passages.

The operation went according to plan with no complications. The patient was nursed on a high dependency bed and made excellent progress during the early post-operative period. He was doing okay except that his abdomen was getting progressively distended due to lack of bowel activity. Since that is not an unusual side effect of major abdominal surgery I decided to continue with expectant treatment in the hope that the paralysed bowel would regain motility.

However, by the eleventh day there was no improvement; abdominal distension was getting worse and Mr D was unable to pass any flatus or faeces through the back passage. Investigations did not point to any mechanical obstruction and there was no immediate indication for surgical exploration. Considering the complex nature of the operation that the patient had, I was quite reluctant to undertake re-exploration unless it was absolutely necessary. At the same time I was getting concerned about the lack of progress, but I was hopeful that the problem would resolve naturally with expectant clinical management. However, with each additional day the intensive care staff and patient's relatives were getting concerned and impatient.

The situation remained unchanged during the next six days. By now the patient was very tired and my intensive care colleagues were becoming increasingly expressive about the need to re-explore the patient's abdomen and decompress the bowel.

It was seventeen days post-surgery. Following a case conference in the morning, I finally agreed to take him back for surgical exploration. However, there was no operating theatre space available on that day. The only time I could undertake the exploratory surgery was late in the evening that day but I decided to postpone it to next day morning for which a theatre slot was available. My team, my anaesthetic colleagues and I had a meeting with Mr D and his family and explained to them the risks of the intended procedure. I also instructed Dr B, a newly appointed senior house officer on duty to inform me immediately if there was any change in Mr D's overall clinical picture.

Dr B was a burly young man of East European origin who had a thick and husky voice and a deep accent. His command of English language was rather patchy.

Late in the afternoon on that drizzly day I walked to the nearby post office to mail an urgent parcel and had to stand for a while in a long line. When my position improved to third in the queue, my mobile phone rang. The caller was none other than Dr B.

"Mr M, this ees Dr B speak-ing, good newz sirr, good newz… Mr D faarrted about 15 minutes before – it was a beeg beeg faarrt – I mean sirr, wind everrywherre on the warrd."

He was quite loud and many people in the queue must have heard what was said. The older lady in front of me tried to control her smile, whereas the younger lady behind me shrugged her shoulders and appeared disgusted with the conversation. I avoided looking around and responded to Dr B by saying, "Okay, I will speak to you later," and turned the phone off quickly.

Keeping my eyes firmly glued to the floor I moved to the service counter, hurriedly handed over the parcel and left. Even though I felt extremely embarrassed, as I left the post office building I looked up into the cloudy sky with a gratifying smile, feeling immensely pleased and relieved that Mr D had turned the corner and would not need another complex major procedure. I went to see him that evening and was delighted to find that the abdominal distension had gone down significantly after he had moved his bowels. The procedure planned for next day was cancelled. He made an uneventful recovery thereafter and many years later he was fit and well. During follow-up consultations he reminded me from time to time about the episode by saying, "Had a narrow escape from your knife Mr M."

Mr D and his beeg beeg faarrt had made my beeg beeg day and gave me a great night's sleep. But that is what a surgeon's world is! Someone flickering his eyes or wriggling her toes, or passing urine, or opening bowels or bringing up a tray-load of smelly phlegm – routine events of day-to-day life, work as tonics, have a tranquilising effect and make a surgeon's day.

In this instance that was a great timing for Mr D – one day made all the difference to him. Had the operating theatre been available on the day, he would have been subjected to another complex surgical exercise. Who knows what would have been the clinical course thereafter? Was it his destiny that shaped events on the day, or was it a mere co-incidence?

That takes me back to the late nineties. On this particular day, I saw Mr A – a sixty two year old, fit gentleman on my ward round in a 6-bedded bay. I had undertaken radical prostatectomy (removal of prostate for cancer) on him the day before. The operation had gone well and he was sitting comfortably in a chair by the first bed in the bay – having tea and toast. He and I had a good conversation about his operation. Following that he stood up, shook my hand firmly and thanked everyone else.

After about fifteen minutes my team and I were with a patient on the fourth bed in the bay when we heard a sudden call for help. Mr A had suddenly become unconscious, the cup had fallen from his hand and the nurse who ran to help him had raised the alarm. We rushed to his bedside and put him on the bed. There was no pulse or heartbeat and he was not breathing either. A cardiac arrest call was sent out, whilst we continued with external cardiac massage. The arrest team took over and after trying cardiopulmonary resuscitation for more than half an hour he was declared dead. Subsequent post mortem examination revealed massive heart attack as the cause of his death.

Everyone was stunned with grief. I continued to feel the firm grip of his right hand for many days thereafter, and could not forget his warm smiling face either. As I write this account I can still see his face and feel his hand. Even today I ask myself the question. Was it his destiny to meet his Creator at the appointed time in the setting described above? There are in fact many incidents with similar themes that come to my mind, and irrespective of one's faith or belief, every clinician would be able to recall clinical episodes where change of circumstances altered the course of events one way or the other. Here is a small selection from other sources.

DATE WITH DESTINY (FROM PN, INDIA, 2005)

I saw a sixty five year old man from a well-known family in the city in the clinic at the teaching hospital where I was working as a consultant. He was suffering from retention of urine due to benign enlargement of prostate. After arranging a series of investigations, including a cardiac assessment I asked the resident staff to get him ready for the operation of transurethral resection of prostate (TURP) on the following Monday afternoon's list. I relayed this information to his daughter who accompanied him. She was well-known locally as a politician and a journalist and she questioned me about the type of anaesthesia that was going to be used.

During the conversation it emerged that her mother had undergone an orthopaedic procedure under spinal anaesthesia and had developed cardiac complications on the operating table allegedly due to the anaesthetic, which according to her had led to her death. Therefore she was keen that her father did not have a spinal anaesthetic. Furthermore, she was highly critical of the orthopaedic surgeon who had operated on her mother and the hospital where the operation had taken place. Despite reminding her politely that surgery and anaesthetic were two different and separate responsibilities, she laid the whole blame for her mother's death on that surgeon and continued to ridicule him during her father's consultation with me.

The patient was admitted to the hospital on Sunday afternoon, the day before the scheduled day of the operative procedure. Two hours after admission he developed sudden chest pain and collapsed. I was called to see him but before me the crash team had already arrived on the scene. Despite timely cardiopulmonary resuscitation, he could not be revived. The cause of death was a fulminating heart attack.

After declaring him dead, on my way home I was naturally sad but I also pondered over the question that instead of Sunday afternoon the cardiac event could have happened twenty four hours later on Monday afternoon – during or soon after prostatic surgery. In that case, until proven otherwise, like the orthopaedic surgeon – who had operated on his wife, I would have been blamed for the catastrophe and would have been the talk of the town. On this occasion a single day made the difference.

Desperate but not dead (WP, UK, 1980)

I was a junior member of the surgical on call team called to the Emergency Department to see a young Japanese student in his early twenties with a knife stuck in his chest. He was alive and clinically stable. He was not in pain but was crying bitterly.

A sad life experience had caused him to attempt ritual suicide but despite his best efforts the knife had glanced off his ribs and lay under the skin in the soft tissues of his chest and upper abdomen. Finding himself alive after the unsuccessful attempt, he had next jumped from a fourth floor window but succeeded only in landing on the soft canvas roof of a passing lorry. His embarrassment was complete when the only surgery that he required was to remove the knife under local anaesthetic, which took only a few minutes; and he was discharged from surgical care soon afterwards. He was clearly destined to live.

Second opinion (PP, USA, 1990)

This happened during the days when radical surgery for localised prostate cancer was not so popular as it is today.

Mr D, a very fit and active sixty eight year old farmer with no associated medical problems, came to my office for a second opinion about the treatment for his cancer prostate that had been diagnosed at a nearby prestigious teaching institution. His wife, and daughter (who was a nurse) accompanied him. But he was reluctant to have an operation because of its potential side effects.

After reviewing his records and after examination, I explained to him and his family all the treatment options available with pros and cons of each treatment. In fact he was already quite knowledgeable about all options anyway.

After listening patiently Mr D responded by saying, "Doctor, I do not want to try any treatment except stilboestrol [female sex hormone] tablets." Stilboestrol was one of the options of treatment used by some surgeons in those days. This was the last option on my list.

His wife and daughter were very unhappy with this particular option and wanted him to follow the advice offered at the hospital, which was to have radical surgery. A loud and vigorous debate between him and his family exploded in my office. I tried my best to calm everyone down. However, Mr B would not settle for anything except the stilboestrol pill.

"You are an obstinate fool – you are destined to die of this cancer," was his wife's opinion.

"I agree with you mum, dad never listened to anyone in his life and he is not listening now. He does not understand; if he wants to kill himself, let him do that," was his daughter's verdict.

The long and turbulent consultation eventually came to a chaotic and inconclusive end, and the trio left my office in a state of total disagreement, shouting and abusing one another.

Many years later Mr B stopped me in a shopping mall. He hadn't changed much and after the pleasantries he reminded me about his visit to my office. "I did not have any treatment for all these years and have not had any problems with my prostate cancer."

"What about your wife and daughter who accompanied you to my office?" I asked curiously.

"My wife had a stroke a year after we saw you and died a few weeks later. My daughter who used to be the nurse died of breast cancer last year." And with a triumphant grin he added, "And they thought I would go first, didn't they?"

The world of Medicine cannot be governed by myths and anecdotes but by scientific evidence and rightly so. However, it is the clinician who puts the evidence into action and executes the final decision on the front line. Guidelines, policies and protocols are there to help but in a number of situations the options are not clear-cut and it is the team leader who makes the final judgment regarding the next course of action, in the best interest of the patient – of course. Such decisions can have far-reaching consequences. In most situations the process is relatively straightforward but sometimes surgeons have to deliberate, consult, research, lose sleep, or even agonise before they make that final call. There are times when they are lost for words and dismiss a bizarre clinical event as a mere coincidence and do no more than brood over the famous quote widely attributed to Albert Einstein that, "Coincidence is God's way of remaining anonymous."

12

WHEN THINGS GO WRONG

Solid body organs (such as the kidney) have a stalk or pedicle that carries the artery or arteries, which supply oxygenated blood to the organ, and the vein or veins that drain deoxygenated blood from the organ. Before removing a diseased or damaged organ the surgeon transects these vessels after obliterating the blood flow through them, usually with thread ties or clips. If the knot slips or a clip opens up, blood will pour out, which can lead to massive haemorrhage with serious consequences. During my early training days I was fascinated by reading the following story about the surgical management of a slipped kidney pedicle in Farquharson's *Text Book of Operative General Surgery*, which used to be the standard textbook on the subject at that time.

A surgeon in France, visited by members of a travelling surgical club, was performing a nephrectomy. One of his visitors recalled the surgeon's reputation for dealing successfully with the problem of the ligature slipping off the renal pedicle. What was the secret? "I will show you," was the reply, as he cut off the kidney with a pair of scissors without first applying either forceps or ligature to the renal vessels. "There is the problem," he said, stuffing large gauze packs tightly into the cavity. He left the operating table, commented on the weather, discussed the political situation and drank a cup of tea. Five minutes passed before he returned to the task. When the packs were gently removed, the field remained dry long enough for him to apply haemostat forceps with great deliberation to both artery and vein. His secret lay in the exercise of restraint, and in allowing sufficient lapse of time for the haemorrhage to be controlled by sustained pressure and reflex vasospasm.'

I read the above story many times and each time wondered how I would deal with a slipped pedicle. I must admit that the very thought of being in that situation made my heart race a bit faster, but I was reasonably confident that the day would never come. However, the day did arrive some years later.

On a late summer afternoon I was about to finish a minor operative procedure on a young boy in one of the two operating theatres at an Iranian hospital, when I was interrupted by one of the theatre personnel who said, "The nurse from the ward has rung to say that the young lady who was operated for nephrectomy (removal of kidney) by Dr N earlier in the day has the drainage bag almost half full with blood. Dr N has left the hospital and we do not know where he is. Should they be doing anything?" I knew that earlier in the day Dr N – a well-respected and highly efficient general surgeon with thirty years experience, had undertaken nephrectomy on a twenty year old girl for an infected, non-functioning kidney.

"After finishing this case I will go up to see her," I replied. The patient was being nursed on the first floor of the hospital not very far from the operating theatre suite, which was situated on the ground floor.

About five minutes later, after finishing my case, as I walked out of the main theatre into the recovery area, the phone rang. One of the theatre nurses picked up the receiver and I could hear the caller screaming desperately for help. "The drainage bag is bursting with blood, what am I going to do – please, please help!"

I raced up the staircase to the room where the patient was admitted. One of the theatre porters – a six-foot tall, broad shouldered man, followed me closely. I could hear his massive body pounding the ground behind me. I found the young lady lying on the bed. She looked whiter than a white rose. A two-litre drainage bag hanging by the bedside was full of blood and looked like a fully inflated red balloon. Her flank was swollen, she was gasping for breath and appeared almost dead. The nurses and other staff were crying and a young man in his twenties was standing nearby with tears rolling down his face. "Quick, let's move her to theatre," I yelled.

Without hesitation, the energetic theatre porter lifted the young lady and her attachments – the tube hanging from the flank connected to a bag and the intravenous drip line that was connected to a bag of normal saline. He ran through the ward, down the stairs and laid her on one of the theatre tables. The anaesthetist who had just finished with my earlier case took immediate charge at the head end of the table. The patient was held on the side and within a couple of minutes I laid the flank wound open, evacuated a massive clot, pushed a large swab in and pressed the swab firmly against the inside of her lumbar spine with my fist. By now she had stopped breathing.

With my fist firmly inside, she was laid flat; the anaesthetist negotiated a tube into her trachea and resuscitation was commenced. After pumping in oxygen, fluids, blood replacement products and blood into her, she perked up and it was pleasing to see her respond successfully. She was then anaesthetised and positioned properly on the side, with my hand still tucked tightly into her belly.

A colleague's fist replaced mine as I got scrubbed. I exposed the kidney bed after taking the swab out carefully. The pulsating renal artery (blood vessel that supplies blood to the kidney) was seen clearly pumping away blood; the vessel was picked easily, clamped and doubly ligated. The wound was closed and the emergency was over. She was transfused a total of twelve units of blood.

Next morning I saw the young lady sitting in her bed eating

breakfast. Her fiancé was sitting close by. As he saw me he got up, hugged me hard and kissed me on both cheeks, one after another (which is the usual custom in the Middle East). He did not speak a word but I could see tears sliding down his face. I found it difficult to hold my own tears.

There were no further complications and she was discharged home after a few days. The couple came to see me before leaving the hospital and invited me to attend their wedding that was scheduled a few months down the line.

I had to tackle an almost similar incident about two decades later in the UK. On that morning one of our senior registrars, who was about to complete the final year of his training and was waiting for a consultant appointment, performed nephrectomy (kidney removal) for cancer on an otherwise fit man in his fifties. The operation had gone well, however, about 12 hours later, just before midnight I received a frenzied phone call from the on call registrar. "Mr M, please come quickly, the patient who underwent nephrectomy earlier today is very poorly. I think the kidney pedicle has slipped."

I rushed from my home to the hospital in my car, the absence of traffic at night helped. The registrar had shifted the patient to theatre, and when I arrived he had already packed the kidney bed. The anaesthetist was pumping blood into the patient to revive his blood pressure. We removed the pack and re-sutured the bleeding vessel without much problem. The patient made an uneventful recovery but the surgeon who was involved with the initial operation was gutted when he heard what had happened.

The surgical encounters described above might sound heroic but the fact is that every surgeon and every member of a surgical team would have a story to tell about a race against time, or a touch and go situation, or a frustrating episode that ended triumphantly. Such situations create a state of intense anxiety and pressure for everyone involved followed by joyous relief once the crisis is tackled successfully. The story described in

Farquharson's book may or may not be true but besides teaching a point of technique it brings home to young surgeons the lesson to remain calm and focussed when confronted with a serious bleeding emergency. Two more real examples from other sources reiterate the same message.

AS COOL AS CUCUMBER (FROM GH, PAKISTAN, 1970)

Mr G was well known for his meticulous surgical technique. He was also a great teacher. On this day he was performing right lumbar sympathectomy for lower limb vascular disease. That used to be a common operation those days and involved making a cut in the flank, finding and removing sympathetic nerve ganglia to interrupt the sympathetic nerve supply to the blood vessels to the lower limb. The expected result was relaxation of the vessel walls and improvement in blood flow to the limb.

Whilst dissecting the sympathetic ganglia, he said to a large audience of juniors and medical students (of whom I was one), "This is where you have to be most careful; you can easily tear one of the lumbar veins that drain directly into the vena cava, and if that happens, the bleeding can be a nightmare. I have seen a patient die on the table after such an accident."

As he repeated the warning, he accidentally tore not one but two of the veins with the result that it started bleeding profusely. This became an emergency situation, as swab after swab became soaked with blood.

For a student beginning his career in medicine this was an alarming experience and since he had warned that the patient could die, the situation was all the more frightening. However, Mr G who was a cool customer by nature and a superb surgeon. He put sustained pressure on the bleeding area for a few minutes, asked for special vascular clamps and carefully applied these to the area, which became dry immediately thereafter. He repaired the torn vena cava, saved the patient and saved the day. This was a live demonstration of what he had been warning about repeatedly and was also a great experience for all present.

THE WALKING WONDER, (FROM PB, UK, 1998)

The incident happened at a private hospital on a late Saturday morning. The first three minor cases had gone well. The fourth and last patient on the list was a lady in her late forties with a tumour arising from the large bowel. She was scheduled to have resection of the diseased part of the bowel by Mr J – a young surgeon about five years into his consultancy who was well respected for his surgical expertise. Everyone in theatre was in a jovial mood, hoping to finish the list by lunchtime.

Mr J opened the abdomen through a midline abdominal incision and the tumour-bearing transverse colon (part of the large bowel) was clearly obvious. The tumour was mobile except the back aspect where it was adherent to the front of the aorta (the main blood vessel running down the centre of abdominal cavity that carries blood from the heart to the lower body). Mr J dissected the tumour off other adjacent structures, and when he finally released it from the aorta there was a 1cm hole on the frontal aspect of the vessel. Blood started gushing in every direction; swab after swab became soaked instantly and there was massive blood loss within minutes.

Mr J kept his nerve and put his right hand inside the abdomen and over a large sponge pushed the aorta hard with his hand against the patient's back thereby blocking the flow through it. Helped by the assistant with his left hand he sucked out the blood and clot and asked for aortic clamps, but there weren't any available at the hospital. There was tension all round!

It took about 45 minutes for a staff member to rush by car to the neighbouring NHS hospital and bring a set of aortic clamps. During all this time Mr J maintained steady pressure on the aorta with his fist, whilst the anaesthetist filled the patient with blood and blood replacement products.

As the clamps were opened from wrappers Mr J released the pressure, applied one clamp above the hole, and another below it, and repaired the defect in the blood vessel with a vascular graft. Thereafter, the diseased segment of colon was removed and bowel continuity re-established. The patient received a total of sixteen units of blood and made an uneventful recovery. She was discharged home on the ninth day and lived an active life for a number of years thereafter. She died of cancer recurrence many years after the original surgical procedure and was well known to every staff member in the hospital. They had nicknamed her 'The Walking Wonder'.

Whilst performing surgical operations under general anaesthetic, one essential member of the team is missing and that is the patient. Of course he or she is there in body – laid out in front of you with the mind drifted away on a cloud of gas, to a land of fantasy where there is no pain. But those of us, who perform the act, have to bear in mind that it is the patient now lost in dreams, who has brought us together, and with whose welfare we are concerned most. And that the person will return – hopefully with improved quality of life. A successful return – which is the norm in the vast majority of cases, makes the whole team happy and proud. The joy is particularly satisfying if the odds are against.

Most surgical episodes end triumphantly, make everyone's day and add colour and weightage to the heroic image of the surgeon and the team involved. The sad reality is that a few – albeit a tiny proportion, conclude on an unhappy note and end in grief, and sometimes in tears.

Ultimate failure – that is loss of life on the operating table is painful for all, even in situations where that is the most anticipated outcome. Commonly they are patients with terrible injuries and the desperate battle by surgical and anaesthetic teams to save life is fought in the operating theatre. I had a brief weeklong experience of working in such a scenario as an emergency surgeon in Ahvaz, Iran at the beginning of the Iraq-Iran war in 1980. Multiple surgical teams were working in makeshift theatres on tens of casualties who were arriving by vanloads. It was tragic to see the ghost of death all round. There was no meaning of life because the boundary between survival and death was blurred; some blamed the carnage to destiny and some described it as collateral damage – and some simply carried on with their work. That week made me realise the meaning and value of life and how hardened military surgeons must become, particularly during an active conflict.

Clinicians witness the end of life on a regular basis but an unforeseen death on the operating table is a terrible tragedy for everyone, in particular for the surgeon. I experienced that not once but twice during my very junior days in the early 1970s. On both occasions the catastrophic event was related to the general anaesthetic. Even though the surgeon had done the job well, in both cases the finger of blame was pointed towards him. In the first case the patient turned blue during the course of a minor surgical procedure that was undertaken under general anaesthetic using an open mask. Much like a driver dozing off behind the wheel a few minutes of lack of concentration on the part of the anaesthetist led to respiratory arrest and attempts to resuscitate were unsuccessful. In the second incident a young man passed away during a routine appendectomy. He practically walked to his death – arrived in the Emergency Department complaining of abdominal pain, was diagnosed as acute appendicitis, walked from the Emergency Department to his bed on the ward and a few hours later from there to the adjacent operating theatre. Subsequent investigation concluded the cause of death to be suxamethonium (succinylcholine) apnoea. The rare condition that was not so well known during those days, occurs when the patient who has been given the muscle relaxant suxamethonium by the anaesthetist prior to surgery, is incapable of metabolising the drug sufficiently rapidly because of an inherited metabolic defect. The individual remains paralysed and cannot regain muscle function quickly enough to be able to breathe spontaneously after the surgery is completed.

On both occasions the day had begun like any other day in the surgical world – in a cheerful and high-spirited manner, but it ended in a disaster. No one could contemplate that the live human lying on the table wouldn't wake up and return back to life. The event was an agonising ordeal for everyone including the surgical and anaesthetic staff. The feeling was that of complete and utter despair – a sense of disbelief overwhelmed by a blanket of darkness, silence and fatigue. Like a personal bereavement you feel the pain but you also implode within with a sense of failure and defeat. Words weren't spoken as thoughts turned to why and what went wrong – and then there was the dread of bringing the news to the family who had handed over their loved one to the clinical team in full faith and with complete trust. The agony lasted for months thereafter.

It must be said that an unexpected death on the operation table is exceedingly rare but not non-existent. Many surgeons and surgical teams are fortunate not to go through a tormenting experience like that during their lifetime. Those who aren't so lucky, have to muster up the courage after the event and carry on. It has been recommended that after such an event the surgical team must stand down for the rest of that day. In my own view they should take some time off.

We surgeons are not supposed to lose patients and sometimes we presume that as long as we do our best, it will come out right in the end. Sadly, that isn't always true!

SELF SUPPLICATION (UK, INDIA 1992)

The hospital where I was working as a registrar at that time received a number of civilian casualties every day due to political troubles in the city. Two operating teams and tables were in readiness round the clock to cater for the injured.

A twenty two year old gentleman was wheeled into the operating theatre during early evening for abdominal exploration. He had received two bullet injuries to his abdomen and was bleeding internally. His family members and relatives were waiting outside the theatre suite. The abdomen was distended and there were two bullet wounds of entry on the abdominal wall, one of which was pouring blood and fluid. The young man was very pale but appeared confident and fully orientated in time and space. He had tachycardia (increased heart rate) and his blood pressure was low. The first person to start proceedings on him was the anaesthetist. "I am going to give you some oxygen. You will need an operation for which we will have to put you to sleep," he said.

The young man's coherent response was, "I know I am not going to live whatever you do. So, please do not bother me."

"Don't say that, you are going to live, you are going to be fine."

"Look, I am telling you, whatever you do, I am going to die," he responded in a firm tone.

The conversation continued with both the patient and the anaesthetist reiterating their respective lines a few times, when the professor (who was the chief surgeon) walked in and came to the anaesthetist's rescue. He caressed the young man's hairy scalp with his right hand and said, "Please calm down my boy. You are going to be fine…"

"You are mistaken sir, I know I am going to die today and I know that for sure."

A number of people tried to convince the young man and after a lot of persuasion he finally gave in and said, "Okay, I will let you put me to sleep on one condition. I want to recite my own funeral prayer before you put that mask on my face."

The deal was agreed. He raised his two supine hands joined together and read the prayer loudly in Arabic, seeking forgiveness for his sins from the Almighty and followed it with recitation of a number of verses from the Holy Quran. As a mark of respect the theatre staff also raised their hands in prayer. It was a very touching and emotional scene.

After the patient was anaesthetised the boss made a midline incision on the abdominal wall. The pressure exerted by the abdominal wall on bleeding vessels eased and blood and clot started gushing out. It became evident that the back wall of abdomen had been shattered by one of the bullets and there was blood pouring from the torn inferior vena cava (the largest blood vessel in the body that carries blood back to the heart) and a number of lumbar veins. Three experienced surgeons and two anaesthetists and a number of assistants and nursing personnel battled for four hours to stop the bleeding and save the young man, but failed. Sadly, he died on the table just before midnight. Everyone was devastated and in tears. The state of bereavement, gloom and shock lasted for many weeks thereafter.

A PERSONAL LOSS (FROM RM, 1970)

This story comes from a provincial hospital in India where I used to work as a house surgeon for Dr K who was the senior surgeon. He was a good surgeon and was well reputed in the area. The patient that he was going to operate on was Mr D, the head of engineering of that province who was equally well known in his field. They had been pals since childhood and had attended the same school and college. After receiving training in the UK in their respective fields both had settled in the same city and had remained close friends throughout their lives. Both were rather overweight and close to retirement.

Mr D was admitted to the hospital the night before the operation. He was a cheerful and chirpy man, and having accomplished all good things in life had no worries of the world. He had a non-functioning kidney that was packed with stones and next day the boss was going to remove the kidney along with the stones. He had undertaken hundreds of such procedures in the past.

Dr K visited Mr D before leaving for home, which was really a social visit because there was no discussion about the impending surgical procedure. "Go to bed early and please skip your night time book for tonight," he advised Mr D.

Mr D was the first case on the list. He was anaesthetised by the senior anaesthetist, positioned and the operative procedure started without any problems. The kidney was quite stuck to the tissues around, but Dr K was his usual self – calm and collected. With masterly technique, the blood vessels supplying the kidney – renal artery and its branches, and renal vein – were dissected neatly. Dr K put a silk ligature around the renal vein and as he tightened the knot the vein was transacted close to its join with the inferior vena cava. Pools of blood started accumulating in the wound. Packs of gauze and pressure failed to stop the blood gushing out. The open vena cava could not be seen. Immediately after removing the pack blood would fill in the wound. Two other surgeons came to help but could not stop the bleeding. After a struggle of two hours Mr D was declared dead on the table.

The theatre was a scene of commotion. Dr K cried like a baby and was inconsolable. Mrs D grabbed Dr K and demanded an explanation; he could do no more than weep bitterly.

Dr K went on leave and announced his retirement a couple of months later. He lost his confidence, his name and his personality. Even though he was physically alive, he had also died with his friend Mr D.

THE DEAD MOTHER (FROM AS, USA, 1992)

I was the consultant on duty for the delivery suite. A charming young lady aged twenty-four was in labour, with her husband sitting by her bedside. Labour was progressing well and it was expected that she would end up having a normal vaginal delivery within a couple of hours. She started complaining of pain in the back and the abdomen, which improved after she had painkillers. However, after a little while the pain returned. There were no abnormal abdominal signs and the baby seemed okay as well. The anaesthetist was asked to administer an epidural for sustained pain relief.

Whilst the anaesthetist was cleaning her back to prepare for the epidural, the patient became confused and crashed suddenly. Her heart and breathing stopped, and the baby became distressed. Whilst she was being resuscitated, I performed an emergency Caesarean section and pulled out a gasping baby from a massive pool of blood. The neonatologists resuscitated the baby successfully. Unfortunately, the mother could not be brought back to life. Despite us trying everything her heartbeat did not return after the crash. She died of abruptio-placentae (premature separation of placenta from the uterus) with amniotic fluid embolism and massive haemorrhage.

Everyone present was shocked and agonised over her death. I could not go back to work for many days. Her sweet face and eyes full of hope would appear in front of me for many months after the sad event. That was undoubtedly the most dreadful experience of my clinical career.

A TRANSPLANT DISASTER (FT, 1980s)

The incident took place at a South Asian teaching hospital where I was working as a junior registrar and affected not one but two people.

A fifty-year old gentleman with chronic renal failure was due to receive a live kidney from his sister who was twenty years younger than him. The chief of surgery was going to remove the donor's kidney in one theatre and a young surgeon who had returned from abroad after training in transplantation was going to transplant the donated kidney into the recipient in the neighbouring theatre. It had taken many weeks to prepare everything; each member of the surgical department – for that matter the whole hospital staff – was excited about the big day because this was the first live donor kidney transplant to be performed at the hospital. The local press had been informed about the event and the news was already in the public domain.

The surgical and anaesthetic teams took up their positions in their respective theatres. The plan was that the donor procedure would commence first and whilst the kidney was being exposed, the operation on the recipient would be started, so that as soon as the kidney was removed from the donor, the recipient would be ready for the new organ transplantation. That would minimise the period of ischaemia (lack of blood supply) time for the transplanted kidney.

I was a junior member of the team in the recipient's theatre waiting alongside others for the recipient to arrive. The transplant surgeon was a jolly character by nature and whilst we were waiting, he was giving us an overview of his interesting experiences of living abroad.

About half an hour after the donor was wheeled into theatre news percolated that there was a serious problem. The endotracheal tube that is normally negotiated into the trachea (wind pipe) to pump oxygen and anaesthetic gas into the patient had been erroneously inserted into the patient's oesophagus (food pipe). Since the patient was fully paralysed with anaesthetic drugs that were administered before the tube was inserted, she was unable to breathe and became blue due to lack of oxygen. The error had only been noticed after a significant time lapse.

All of us rushed to the donor theatre, where another anaesthetic colleague had just managed to negotiate an endotracheal tube into the windpipe. Everyone was on tenterhooks, hoping that once the oxygen was pumped in, the patient would recover. All surgeons and anaesthetists – senior as well as junior – and nursing staff were praying for her recovery.

However, that was not to be. After remaining in coma for many days the donor died. There was distress and devastation all round. The hospital and surgeons became the subject of rebuke in the local press and the anaesthetist was dismissed. It was a sad week in the history of a famous hospital in that part of the world. The transplant programme suffered a serious set back, and it was many years before it was reinvigorated.

The recipient continued on dialysis but died of an inter-current complication a couple of months after the incident.

The lay press remains on the look out and publishes dramatic stories about surgical mishaps on a regular basis. In some cases the content is exaggerated but the sad fact is that adverse surgical events do happen even in the best hospitals in the world. These range from surgical flow interruptions to minor accidents to catastrophic events. Even though the majority of such incidents happen within the operating theatre environment, some errors occur or take root well before the patient enters the theatre suite.

Time is of the essence when dealing with a serious incident in the operation theatre. This is particularly so if it is due to an anaesthetic error – a few minutes of compromised airway can have catastrophic or even fatal consequences like in the examples described before. On the other hand surgeons have relatively more time to rectify a surgical mistake and that gives them the space to seek help from colleagues within and outside their own specialty if required. Provided that the complication is recognised and rectified during the course of the primary procedure the outcome is generally good.

As a member of the appointments panel for many consultant surgeon appointments, I frequently asked candidates to recount any alarming theatre episodes they witnessed during their training years. I heard a number of answers but the most worrisome included: a surgeon hammering an inappropriate size intra-medullary nail into a transversely fractured femur resulting in longitudinal shattering of the bone; drilling too deep during surgery on the spine and driving the drill into the aorta, damaging the front wall of inferior vena cava (main vein draining blood from lower body to heart) during excision of right kidney and removal of part of the urinary bladder during a caesarean section.

Injury to an adjacent organ or structure is, however, the commonest surgical complication. Examples include common bile duct (tube draining bile from liver to bowel) injury during gall bladder surgery; perforation of bowel during laparoscopic surgery; bleeding from the spleen or liver during abdominal surgery, damage to ureter (tube connecting kidney to bladder) during gynaecological or pelvic surgery and damage to a large blood vessel in the vicinity of the surgical field. The last one can lead to rapid blood loss with risk of death.

In many instances the inadvertent injury is the result of a difficult anatomical terrain, but in a small minority, wrong technique, lack of attention to detail, carelessness, lack of experience, tiredness or haste by surgeons or their teams are the causative factors. And that can happen even with common and/or minor procedures. One of my senior trainees removed too much foreskin whilst circumcising a child with the result that the child had to be transferred straightaway to a plastic surgery centre with an open penile wound. On investigation it was clear that it was not due to lack of training or knowledge, but due to a temporary lapse of concentration during the procedure.

Speeding is the most important and the commonest cause of a road traffic accident. The statement is equally pertinent in surgical practice where hurrying can cause damage and lead to suffering and pain. Despite stringent driving tests that examine and assess an individual under test conditions there are still a few drivers who are skilful and well trained but they get a kick from speeding and end up with a disastrous crash. Surgery is no different – roadside warnings on the highways such as, *speed thrills but kills* and *speed is knife that cuts life* are applicable to all aspects of surgical practice.

TIDY IT UP OLD CHAP (*TT, UK, 1970*)

The incident took place before the keyhole surgery era, when gall bladders were removed by an open operation. I was then a senior registrar and was working in the next theatre while the boss was performing an open cholecystectomy (removal of gall bladder) in the main theatre. He was a slick surgeon but was always in a hurry and rushed everyone. The registrar and the senior house officer were helping him. The latter had joined the unit recently. He was quite experienced because he had worked in general surgery for a number of years in his home country. Being the second assistant he was standing on the surgeon's side of the table holding a retractor and could not see what was going on.

The boss quickly dissected and ligated the duct and blood vessels connected to the gall bladder and turning to the senior house officer he said, "Tidy it up old chap." In the same breath he said to the registrar, who was the first assistant, "Let's go and quickly see that patient on the ward." With that both the boss and the registrar left the operating theatre in a flash. The senior house officer along with the house officer who scrubbed to help, were left to "tidy up".

After about forty-five minutes the boss and the registrar returned to theatre at the same time as the patient was being wheeled out into the recovery area.

"How did it go?" he asked the senior house officer.

"Quite okay." he replied confidently.

"Did you remove the gall bladder?"

"No, I just closed the abdomen, I thought you had removed it."

"I had released and cut the vessels and the duct. All you

had to do was to dissect the gall bladder from the liver bed and remove it." he replied angrily.

"Err – I am really sorry, I thought, you…"

The boss yelled, "Wheel her back to theatre."

The patient was put to sleep again, the wound was reopened, the gall bladder was removed and the wound closed again.

A RECLESS MOMENT (GB, UK, *1984*)

A senior registrar awaiting a consultant appointment joined the surgical unit where I was working as a senior house officer. He was bright, fast and furious and had a skilful pair of hands. He was so quick that assistants and scrub nurses were unable to keep pace with him. He would often boast, "There is no scrub nurse who can put up with my speed." The words, "please don't rush me" were often heard from nurses who helped him.

One day he started cholecystectomy (open removal of gall bladder) on a lean lady in her mid-thirties. He made a deep, long and oblique cut on the abdomen below and parallel to the rib margin. Since the liver edge was a few centimetres below the margin his cut went through her liver slicing a chunk of it off. There was blood everywhere; she needed a massive blood transfusion. Eventually she came off the table alive after six hours toil by three senior surgeons, following which she was transferred to a tertiary care centre where she had to battle out one complication after another. After many months of hospital stay she was eventually discharged.

The speedster probably learnt his lesson at the expense of anguish, pain and suffering of another human being.

Some surgical incidents have been designated by the Department of Health in England as 'Never Events'. This means they are so serious they should never happen in a healthcare setting. These include retained foreign bodies like surgical swabs, wrong site/side surgery and wrong implant/prosthesis – all preventable surgical blunders. NHS England reported 290 and 312 Never Events in 2012-2013 and 2013-2014 respectively. In both years >80% of such events fell into one of the three aforementioned categories.

Mainly due to the introduction of stringent checks and balances the incidence of mistakes in swab and instrument counting after surgical operations has declined markedly in recent years. Regrettably, such incidents are still reported from time to time. Thankfully none of my patients was ever re-explored to recover a missing swab or a surgical instrument, although I am aware of three such incidents that happened in the organisations where I worked during my lifetime. However, I recall an incident in my own practice when the scrub nurse stopped me from closing the abdomen because the swab count was short by one. I launched an extensive search of the abdominal cavity but could not find the missing swab. X-ray of the abdomen failed to show the swab but the nurses were adamant that the swab count was not correct. All bins were searched but the lost swab could not be found. It was a frustrating dilemma for all. As I started deliberating with managers and colleagues about our next line of action a student nurse found a discarded surgical latex glove rolled like a ball inside a theatre bin. The glove felt spongy, so she laid it open and discovered the missing swab inside the infolded glove. I remembered instantly that at the beginning of the surgical operation as I wiped the excess antiseptic from the skin with a dry swab, my sterile gloved hand touched an unsterile surface. I therefore removed the glove from my hand and in doing so inverted it. The swab that was in my hand, remained inside the glove. No one present in theatre saw me doing this and the glove along with the sponge within it was binned. I was the culprit responsible because I forgot all about it. Amidst scenes of joyous relief I had to hide my blushes, accept my error, and apologise.

Bringing a patient back to theatre for re-exploration to recover a missing swab or instrument is a surgical calamity for the whole theatre team and the hospital, and a personal tragedy for the scrub nurse and the surgeon. Such an incident is also a shocking setback for the patient and the family members. In the bizarre story that follows the patient underwent a second operation to remove a missing (mislaid!) swab.

MY SWAB COUNT WAS CORRECT! (KM, IRAN, 1978)

The incident happened during the nineteen eighties at a teaching hospital where I was working as a resident. A lady in her early thirties underwent routine abdominal hysterectomy (removal of uterus). The initial post-operative period was fine but after the second day she started having a high temperature with progressive abdominal distension. A plain abdominal X-ray revealed a radio-opaque shadow resembling a swab in the centre of the abdomen.

The nurse who had scrubbed for the operation had an unblemished theatre career spanning over twenty years. She was devastated to hear the news but pleaded strongly that all swabs had been accounted for. However, the chief who had performed the operation, and the radiologist who reported on the x-ray, were of the opinion that a swab was inside the abdomen. The patient was therefore taken back to theatre for abdominal exploration.

The wound was reopened and the abdominal cavity searched, but no swab was found. The distended bowel was delivered outside the abdomen and a second search launched but the swab could not be found. The theatre atmosphere became tense as frustration over the inability to find the swab mounted. A fellow gynaecology consultant colleague also got scrubbed and explored the abdominal cavity but the swab was not seen or felt anywhere. By now the patient had been on the table for more than three hours. No one could understand the mystery of the missing swab.

At this point a young trainee anaesthetist walked into theatre. After becoming aware of what was happening, she mustered the courage to ask the question, "Sir, did this lady have a spinal anaesthetic for hysterectomy?"

"Yes, she did," was the reply from one of the gynaecology juniors who was assisting with the operation.

"Did you look at her back? The swab may be covering the skin at the site where the spinal needle went in."

The wound was covered with a large swab and the lady was turned on her side. Lo and behold – the swab was sitting right there on the lumbar spine, fixed to skin with strips of surgical tape. There were emotional scenes in theatre. Everyone was happy that the swab had been found but there was sadness that the lady had an unnecessary second major operation. The chief was utterly disappointed about the dreadful mistake, but the scrub nurse who had assisted in the first operation cried with delight, saying repeatedly, "My swab count was correct."

Wrong site or side surgery is another surgical blunder that must never happen. Such an event devastates the surgeon and destroys the reputation of the department and the hospital. For the patient and the family it is an unforeseen calamity. Nonetheless reports of such errors continue to trickle from all over the world. Of the 306 'Never Events' recorded in the UK from 1 April 2014 to 31 March 2015, 124 were of wrong side surgery.

In recent years healthcare organisations in the West have invested heavily into risk management systems. Since the establishment of National Patient Safety Agency in the UK in 2001 a lot of effort has been devoted to entrench the principles of safety and quality into the tributaries of healthcare organisations, within and outside the NHS. It must be said that a lot of headway has been achieved but it is still work in progress and an on-going process.

Major determinants and mechanisms of failure that culminate in a 'Serious Incident' (SI) or a 'Never Event' or a 'Near Miss' include system factors, human factors and team factors. Having worked as a senior healthcare manager and having been involved in professional and organisational regulation and in the investigation of serious incidents in healthcare, in my experience poor systems and inefficient processes are the usual causes of failure. A minor error carried along a chain ends up in a major catastrophe.

Human factors are also an important determinant of failure. Fatigue, stress and anger on the part of the surgeon or the anaesthetist can translate into wrong decisions and actions. Sometimes the insight to acknowledge the need to seek help from a colleague is lacking. The clinician involved may not have the competence or expertise of undertaking a procedure and instead of seeking help may still have a go. The Hippocratic Oath (modern version) is clear in this regard and stipulates that; *'I will not be ashamed to say "I know not," nor will I fail to call in my colleagues when the skills of another are needed for a patient's recovery.'* And so too is the GMC document 'Good Medical Practice' (2013) which specifies that, *'You must recognise and work within the limits of your competence.'*

In the surgical environment it is important to have clear lines of responsibility and good leadership. A disorganised and free for all operating theatre is a fertile ground for misadventure. At the same time a steep authority gradient – which used to be prevalent in the surgical world in the past, doesn't allow a junior member of the team to point out an error that's about to occur. That is what happened at the Welsh hospital – the medical student watching the operation tried unsuccessfully to warn the surgeon that he was removing the wrong kidney.

Surgical mishaps not only hurt the patient but also friends, loved ones, and family members. There is dismay, frustration and suffering when things go wrong. You feel let down and the bond of trust between the giver and recipient of care evaporates instantly. Such events also shatter surgeons' and surgical teams' morale and destroy confidence. Some end up with coroners' inquests and some lead to compensation claims. A few have recently culminated in criminal prosecutions but many end up as Fitness to Practise hearings.

The clinical governance framework introduced in the UK in 1998 made healthcare organisations 'accountable for continually improving the quality of their services and safeguarding high standards of care by creating an environment in which excellence in clinical care will flourish'. It is now a routine in the UK and US for healthcare providers to report key performance indicators of safe surgical practice such as: surgical complication rates, returns to operating theatre, readmission rates and so on. The quantitative analysis of clinical outcome parameters like the Hospital Standardised Mortality Ratio (HSMR) and Summary Hospital-level Mortality Indicator (SHMI) made it possible to benchmark healthcare providers and clinicians – in particular surgeons. These measures helped to inculcate the concepts of patient safety within the mind-sets of healthcare staff.

Steps to prevent 'Never Events' have been instituted in western hospitals, with structured communication between the patient, the surgeon(s), anaesthetist(s) and other members of the healthcare team. It is now compulsory for hospitals to verify the surgical procedure to be performed and mark the surgical site in advance. The drill of using the World Health Organisation (WHO) Surgical Safety Checklist in operation theatres has become a mandatory practice. It is also a routine to take the "Time Out" prior to starting an operation when team members discuss the patient and prepare themselves for any potential problems that might arise during the procedure. Despite being a monotonous, boring and repetitive exercise this has been a great leap forward in patient safety agenda. The practice needs to be propagated and implemented worldwide.

13

GRATITUDE AND TRUST

It is quite common in the land of my birth for patients and their relatives to express gratitude to their care provider by saying, "God has blessed you with *dast-i-shifa* [healing hand]." In Iran the linguistic delicacy of Persian language takes the conversation to a different level of imagination. After finishing a surgical procedure the surgeon is routinely greeted by patients, relatives and even staff with one of the following expressions: *"Dast-i-shuma dard na kunae"*, which translates to: "Hope your hand doesn't ache", or *"Khasta na baashee"*, meaning "Hope you are not feeling tired". These lingoes are part of everyday exchange in the operating theatre. In the West, thank you cards and letters of appreciation for the surgeon and the team arrive on a regular basis. Some of the expressions are very flattering and carefully thought out. Some arrive even after a patient's demise and can be quite tender and touching. Here are a few chosen from a large bunch of thank you letters from my own collection, the first from the daughter of a lady and the other two from grateful spouses:

"... mum thought the world of you, she often mentioned the hug you gave her when she was very down and in some way that was more important than the drugs she was given..."

"Thank you for looking after her so well. You gave her almost seven years more life, and she went out like a butterfly on a summer day."

"… and you fought very hard to keep him alive, God bless you and your family."

Once in a while patients or their close family members show their indebtedness by offering lyrical tributes and showing off their poetic talents. The following is a copy of a letter penned by the wife of one of my patients in 2002.

My Gucci Bag

A reluctant acquisition!
But needs must
So on best recommendation
had to have it!
Very exclusive, and precious
Hand crafted… Designer made!
"Green" … But not in colour,
Made from recycled materials
No pockets, belts or flaps
Perfectly hand stitched and functional
With every minute detail considered
Uniquely made for me
Bespoke even!
And absolutely priceless
No… not a fashion accessory…
My Neo-bladder
My life!

A Neo-bladder (new bladder) is created from the loops of patient's own bowel after the removal of the diseased (usually cancerous) urinary bladder, which is then joined with the normal urethra (water-passage) to re-route the flow of urine.

Another patient of mine sent the following poem that describes the experiences of his hospital stay.

Raising A Toast

Now what about the night shift, no witches ghosts or ghouls
But cuddly mama D will protect us from such fools
In the depths of night if you listen strange squiggles you will hear
It is jolly J the "T" line a practising I fear
And hail to saucy S, she is really quite a bird
She towers above you with a hypo, but your screams are never heard
As sexy c – stalks the ward she is the prostate patient's perk
With flashing lights at 4am, and the sleeping pills don't work

At last it is the technics team, with lasers knives and string
They cut you open, stitch you up, by God it don't half sting
First Dr S J at blood she doesn't faint
With M always by her side, she is accompanied by a "saint"
And Dr "Hot Lips" R his energy never sags
In and around theatre he tears around in drag

And lastly to my surgeon Mr M and his merry men
I must not sound too frivolous or they'll have me in again
My thanks to all those people, who do their jobs so well
I raise and toast your health, in my book you all are swell

A UK colleague was kind enough to share this poem that he received from one of his grateful patients.

The Prostate Man!

When your prostate goes down the pan
don't you worry I know a man
Because everybody needs a jolly good man
when that worn out prostate goes down the pan.

It was my good luck to find him quick
when my PSA went lickety spit.
Well what do you do and know 'bout these things unseen?
Prostates are part of your dreams.

Did you know that without that thing you wouldn't be here
Mate – nor would the queen.
Reproduction, it's true, is a vital part
of a universe that started with a gigantic f**t.

Oh, I am sorry my dear I got carried away
I'm just so relieved to be here today.
Do you want to know now the name of my man?
What else would it be but "Mr…!"

Yes Mr… is the prostate man
and he whips 'em out just as fast as he can.
With a little snip here and a snip there,
a polythene bag and a wing and a prayer

WHOOSH, you cannot even feel a thing
and that prostate is history, ring a ding ding.

Some convey the message by showing off their artistic talents. On a preoperative appointment before having an operation on his prostate, one of my patients brought with him a picture drawn by him, of an older looking languid man, with a dripping tap attached to his nether region, being walked to the operating theatre by two stern looking nurses. When I asked him how he felt, he replied, "Mr M, the picture says it all!"

Large donations to medical charities and charitable organisations and medical institutions are a routine phenomenon in the West. Of the smaller gifts, chocolates and sweets are the most favoured item and it is not unusual for patients to bring along a bottle of wine or champagne as tokens of gratitude. Sometimes these items are delivered as Christmas presents.

Offering live gifts to their carers is quite common in small towns and villages in South Asia. These can include a cockerel or a hen; and if the patient belongs to a well-to-do family, even a sheep or a goat.

Some patients put in a lot of effort into the choice of a present; one of my patients brought me a key chain from Brussels that was a miniature replica of the famous Brussels' *Manneken Pis figurine* – the bronze statue of a young boy urinating. She thought that was an appropriate item for a urological surgeon. Another patient, who undertook woodcarving as a hobby, carved a small bird in oak with his name inscribed on its base. He died soon after but the present has been part of my office table furniture for more than two decades. Sometimes gifts arrive in unexpected circumstances.

Accompanied by his wife, a smartly dressed banker in his forties came to see me complaining of a scrotal lump. After I examined him suddenly he turned pale, went into a state of panic and almost passed out. It took him a few minutes to recover after which his first comment was, "Is it cancer? I want you to be honest with me, please."

"It could be, but we need to arrange a scan urgently – and even if that is the case the overall prognosis of testicular tumours is excellent," I replied uneasily.

He got up slowly, put on his shirt and trousers and sat back in the chair in front of me and said, "Normally I am quite calm and take things in my stride but on this occasion I lost my composure for which I apologise."

I had a lengthy conversation with him and his wife about the diagnosis and the need for urgent investigations and at the end offered my apologies. "It was probably my body language that gave it away," I admitted.

And then there was silence for a while whilst he started unrolling his tie carefully, which he had rolled equally carefully before he had got undressed. In order to break the embarrassing gap in conversation and to lighten up the atmosphere I remarked, "That is a nice tie!"

"Err! Do you like it?" he said smilingly.

I chose not to answer.

The scan confirmed the diagnosis of a testicular tumour following which he underwent a surgical procedure. He returned for the first follow up consultation a week later and as he sat in the chair he handed over to me a thank you card and a boxed present and asked me to open it. Inside was a replica of the tie that I had commented about during our first meeting.

I thanked him profusely. He responded by saying, "I hope you like it. This will remind you about my squeamish behaviour. But thank you for sorting me out so quickly. I guess you had to tell me the truth – sooner the better!"

I opened the card after they left. The writing inside read, "Please accept this small gift. This is nothing compared to what you helped me with – – – the precious gift of life. With love & regards…"

It is certainly not the gift that matters but the thought behind it. If offered with love it is heart warming and priceless.

OMELETTE FOR BREAKFAST (FROM AH, BANGLADESH, 2009)

My wife (who is a nurse) and I are based in the UK. We took up a short-term charity assignment in the northwest of Bangladesh to work at a mobile floating hospital. The hospital was open to the general public but a patient had to get registered before being seen by a doctor. The registration fee was five takas (about three British pennies) per patient.

One day it was brought to my attention that one of the men who had brought his wife for consultation could not afford to pay the registration charge. I instructed that the fee should be waived and after a while in came a middle-aged gentleman along with his wife of a similar age. After examination I prescribed her the appropriate medication, which was supplied free of charge. The couple were profusely thankful when they left.

Two days later the gentleman returned with two eggs, which had been laid by their family hen. He refused to leave until my wife and I accepted the gift. After agreeing rather reluctantly to his first request, he made a second request and would not leave until he had witnessed my wife and I consuming the eggs. This was an unusual request but his persuasiveness was so intense that we had no other choice but to say yes. We cooked an omelette with some ghee, salt and chillies and ate it in his presence.

Gratitude can be shown in other forms too – like being allocated a better seat for a theatre show, being presented with hospitality seats for a sports event and so on but sometimes you are dumbfounded by an act of goodwill from unexpected quarters especially when you are in a tight corner.

A FRIEND IN NEED (FROM BK, UK, *1976*)

During my early training in obstetrics, well before the widespread usage of debit and credit cards, and cash point machines, I took up a senior house officer post at a county hospital in England. After a couple of weeks of hectic duties I managed to find some time to go to a bank to withdraw some cash. The counter clerk asked me to fill in a cash withdrawal form, which I did. As I handed over the form to him, the conversation went something as follows:

"Can I see your ID please?" he said.

"I am sorry I do not have any ID with me."

"Can you show me the proof of your address please?"

"I have no address yet, I live in a single accommodation at the local hospital."

"Okay, show me the proof of being an employee at the hospital."

"I am so sorry, I don't have that either." I said rather sheepishly.

"I am sorry doctor, I can't give you any money." He replied with a whiff of authority.

I started pleading, but he wouldn't budge. A couple of individuals standing in the front portion of the queue behind me were getting restless because of the wait and started advising me to get the ID and come back. As I was about to leave the counter a lady in the back of the queue shouted, "I am his ID. I know him very well."

A pretty and elegantly dressed woman in her middle thirties stepped forward to the counter and said to the clerk, "I can certify to you that he is a doctor and works at the hospital – actually he helped me to deliver a beautiful baby last Monday. If that does not convince you, I will withdraw money from my own account for the doctor and take it from him later. Mind you, I have my ID with me."

That satisfied the clerk and I got the cash, which was debited to my account.

PAYBACK TIME (FROM KP, INDIA, 1968)

This incident dates back to the era when the only imaging technology available was an x-ray. This was my first job as a junior resident at a 600-bed hospital. Master L, a three-year old child was admitted as an emergency with head injury. The parents were on a holiday and were staying in a hotel room on the second floor, which was connected to a balcony. The child had apparently walked to the balcony without the parents noticing and fell on the road in the main street. He was immediately rushed to the local hospital where I was working as an intern and was the first on call.

On admission Master L was deeply comatose and on examination there was one centimetre laceration on the scalp covered with what looked like brain tissue. I cleaned the wound, applied a fresh dressing, and after discussion with the boss the child was kept under observation.

He was an only child and had been born after twelve years of wedlock. The parents were totally devastated and in a state of panic. He remained in a coma for more than a week and I visited him many times during that period. I would sit by the child's bedside and chat with the parents. On the eighth day all of a sudden he started moving his body and within the next couple of days he woke up. To everyone's delight he recovered completely and was discharged from the hospital with no neurological deficit or disability.

His parents were enormously grateful to me. Erroneously they believed that I was somehow instrumental in his recovery. His father, who was a jeweller by trade, gave me his postal address and invited me to visit his place, which was about 700 miles away. I had no intention of doing that but I noted the address in my diary.

Many years later I was about to begin a thirty-hour train journey from one Indian city to another. Just after embarking the train at a crowded railway station, in a flash my bag (with all my belongings including my wallet) was stolen. No sooner did I realise that my bag was gone the train started moving and I was left with nothing except my diary and some loose change which wasn't enough even for one meal – I was in a serious difficulty!

A couple of hours later – whilst I was still in a state of shock, the train stopped at an intermediate railway junction where the stoppage time was one hour. It suddenly dawned on me that the train would also be stopping at the place where Master L's parents lived. Luckily I spotted the post office at the station and using the loose change I sent a telegram to Master L's dad informing him that I would be visiting him and would arrive by train at the scheduled time.

Just after midnight the train pulled into the station where Master L's parents lived. Through the train window I could see the bald head and the short and round figure of Master L's dad standing on the platform, accompanied by a large welcoming party. Soon after exchanging pleasantries he asked me, "Where is your luggage Dr P?"

Hesitatingly I replied, "You mean my luggage! That should arrive tomorrow –I hope."

After boarding the car with Master L's parents I narrated my story to them. The father had a big laugh and advised me to relax. He was not interested in my story but was only keen to tell me how well his son was. After a hearty meal I went to bed, and next morning at breakfast I mustered the courage to say to Master L's dad, "Can I borrow some money, sir?"

After a paroxysm of laughter he responded by saying, "I will have to think about that," and the conversation ended there.

A couple of hours later he asked me to follow him to a room in the basement of his house. There was a massive safe standing in one corner of the room. After turning a few keys he opened the safe and said in a very soft voice, "Please take what you want," and after speaking those words he left the room. To my utter disbelief I found myself standing in front of an open safe stuffed with jewellery, gold, silver and bundles of cash. I felt very nervous partly because I had never seen so much wealth before and partly for the reason that there was no one else in the room. I sat down and waited for the arrival of my host, who turned up about twenty minutes later – this time accompanied by his wife.

"Did you take what you wanted?"

"No, I didn't," I said meekly.

"I left the safe open so that you could choose whatever you needed… it would be our greatest pleasure if you did that."

I was overwhelmed and simply asked for a sum of money that would take me comfortably to my destination.

"Okay, if that is what you wish – that is fine with us." And he handed over to me a sum of money and closed the safe door. A few weeks later I sent the borrowed amount back to him by postal money order, which he declined to cash and returned it with a curt message.

Every clinician would be able to recount generous gestures in various forms from ex-patients. A UK colleague remembered visiting a patient on the ward on whom he had performed an emergency operation the night before. By her bedside was sitting the manager of a world famous English football club. He didn't know him but the lady patient introduced the two to each other. Two days later the surgeon received a parcel containing two club shirts signed by the manager and a football signed by all players. He left all these goods in the loft space of his house. Twenty years later while clearing the junk he found them and gifted one to his 30-year old son who was a member of that club. Little did he know that the shirt was then worth a fortune. In the interest of fairness he gifted the other shirt to his second son. He didn't tell me what he did with the football?

I had my quota of generosity too. For instance I received an early warning e-mail from a patient's wife informing me about the date of impending sales at a well-known UK department store – where she worked as a senior manager.

A few years ago, I was travelling in economy class on a long-haul overseas flight and was intensely absorbed with my Sudoku puzzle. Suddenly I felt a gentle tap on my right shoulder – it was the cabin director who was my ex-patient. The gentleman was a loud character by nature and as I raised my head he showered at me a noisy welcome – he blurted out my name and within a few minutes the sparsely populated cabin knew that I was a surgeon and had treated him in the past. Thankfully he didn't divulge the details of why he had consulted me. The whole cabin's gaze focused on me. I felt so embarrassed and after he left I kept my head down and acted as if I was totally absorbed with my reading material. A few minutes later, while I was still recovering from my blushes one of the airline attendants approached me and said in a feeble tone, "I have been asked to direct you to your new seat." As I started shuffling from my seat, once again all eyes converged on me. However, without looking at anyone I disappeared from the scene and found myself occupying a seat in the business class cabin.

Sickness is an adversity that a patient has to deal with and transforming an adversity into a success story brings the greatest satisfaction to the surgical soul. The patient paints that story into a lovely picture known as gratitude, which not only makes a surgeon's day but also transforms routine surgical jobs into sheer joy. Compliments and commendations in all forms and shapes are like music to your ears. They are particularly comforting when they appear to be genuine and sincere. Like everyone else surgeons too have feelings and emotions. They too feel good when praised by patients and their loved ones, colleagues and peers. Appreciation helps them to unwind and feel contented with what they do. It encourages them to improve their performance and bolster their achievements. For a surgeon as well as the patient the final determinant of success and satisfaction is of course the quality of care offered and the end result of treatment.

Mark Twain said, "I can live for two months on a good compliment." I would say that compliments live with you forever.

I still remember with fondness the compliment by Prof K after I put a row of skin sutures on his patient. That was my date with my destiny. If I acquired the power to press the rewind button and go back in time to that day, I would love to have the same conversation with him and his theatre assistant again. The truth is that I wouldn't hesitate even for a moment to start all over again.

14

POSTSCRIPT

"It is not the strongest of the species that survive,
nor the most intelligent,
but the one most responsive to change."
— Leon C Megginson

I have been enormously lucky to travel across the length and breadth of the surgical Masaai Mara for more than forty years. I observed its dusks and dawns, mingled with its inhabitant creatures and a vast number of its visitors, felt comforted and energised by its abundant warmth, enjoyed its action-packed adventures, reflected over its melancholic moments and saw its tributaries expand and branch out. Surgery fed me with successes that kept me blooming, pumped me up with unexpected triumphs that made me wonder, challenged me with surprises that made me strong, bogged me down with sorrows that taught me the meaning of failure and made me feel humble and in trusting acceptance of God's will. Surgery is not for the weak minded or the faint hearted, and is certainly not for the rash and the reckless.

My training years shaped the foundation of my building, which was slowly constructed brick by brick over my working lifetime. During my journey, science and technology progressed at an unbelievable pace, and with that, my own building underwent many architectural alterations, extensions and design modifications. A number of ground breaking scientific inventions changed the whole profile of surgical art and craft. Like a suspenseful mystery played on the stage, one scene replaced another, as old concepts were laid to rest and new ones became a routine. To shun the familiar and long-standing notions and practices was difficult; to learn and accept the new ones was equally so. On reflection I feel I have been a witness as well as a part of an incredible fairy tale, in which fiction and fantasy of yesterday transformed into factual reality of today, before my very own eyes.

I smelt the surgical air at a time when – in the villages and many urban areas of my land of birth, Kashmir – barbers and paramedical personnel circumcised male children, drained abscesses and plucked out loose teeth; wise elderly women controlled some of the midwifery practice, and bonesetters enjoyed a lucrative trade. At that time the world had recovered fully from the hangover of the greatest surgical invention of all time – Joseph Lister's epic discovery of the concept of antisepsis – that had been complemented a few decades later by Fleming's discovery of penicillin – the wonder drug capable of killing bacteria. Courtesy of these two famous people, the surgeon was equipped with smart weapons to prevent and treat infection – the deadly foe that had killed countless humans in the days gone by. Both these inventions, which germinated in mainland Britain, had transformed the surgical landscape all over the world, and as a surgical toddler, I had the luxury of prescribing and administering penicillin and its broad-spectrum variants freely and in full dosage to my patients. The quest was on to find more antibiotics – stronger, faster acting and with broader efficacy against different bacteria. With time it became difficult for the medical fraternity to keep pace with new names – any new drug with the suffix 'in' was an antibiotic unless proven otherwise.

The clinician assumed that antibiotics were not only the

answer to all infective problems of mankind, but also a shortcut to good surgical practice. However, within thirty years, by the time I had mellowed into a senior hospital surgeon and healthcare manager, bacteria had become smart enough to develop defence mechanisms against antibiotics as overuse of these drugs led to bacterial resistance. The seriousness of this threat was conveyed in the grim warning by England's Chief Medical Officer in her 2013 Annual Report: *'Global action is needed to tackle the catastrophic threat of antimicrobial resistance, which in twenty years could see any one of us dying following minor surgery.'*

To make matters worse, clinicians and health planners were confronted with another challenge: indiscriminate prescribing resulted in the growth of rogue bacteria like methicillin resistant staphylococcal aureus (MRSA) and clostridium difficile (C Diff), which started invading the human space. The modern surgeon had to revisit the techniques of proper hand washing and pay attention to antisepsis, something that our predecessors had followed like religious commandments in the decades gone by.

It was initially hard for surgeons to go back to basics, but they had no choice; wide media coverage with good evidence highlighted infection as a serious threat to patient safety. Scrutiny and regulatory framework had also exposed the failures and inadequacies of surgical systems and the disparities in surgical outcomes amongst surgeons and organisations. Benchmarking of quality indicators amongst surgeons and healthcare providers slowly transformed the surgical landscape in the West. Effective regulation, multi-disciplinary decision making, appraisal methodologies involving feedback from patients, peers and line managers, coupled with widely published displays of validated outcomes like mortality rates and ratios, complication and readmission rates, and other information tools educated patients and the public about what to expect from a healthcare provider. It also changed the ways of thinking of surgeons, and the overall cultural landscape of surgery.

The present day surgeon is fully aware of the various systems that help to drive the patient safety agenda and the delivery of high quality care. However, in order for the systems and processes to become effective tools, these need to be owned and led by clinicians and not by inexperienced and overzealous managers. Furthermore, patient safety can only be improved in a true no-blame culture, in which each error and each compliment is treated as an opportunity to learn and to improve clinical care. A surgeon with the threat of blame hanging on his neck will be loath to take a chance in a high-risk surgical setting. Whilst we identify, debate and wherever possible minimise failures by learning from them, we need to celebrate successes and achievements of surgeons and surgery.

At the dawn of my surgical existence various anaesthetic agents were already in use, and the control of airways with tubes placed into the trachea had already been perfected. Surgery was no longer a painful torture that I had witnessed as a child. The anaesthetic specialty was, however, still in its infancy in many parts of the world and the staffing levels were very low. The pouring of flammable ether liquid on to the facemask of a struggling victim by medical personnel not trained in anaesthetics was not an uncommon sight. A patient would routinely comment: "I am not afraid of the operation, but I am scared that I may not wake up."

The surgeon viewed the anaesthetist at best as a junior associate – a member of the team whose job was to keep the patient quiet whilst the head craftsman performed the handiwork on the subject. The unequal relationship was reflected at the highest level; for instance, in the UK the Faculty of Anaesthetists that was founded in 1948 functioned within the patronage of the Royal College of Surgeons of England. The faculty became the College of Anaesthetists in 1988 but still remained a college within a college until 1993 when it acquired complete independence as the Royal College of Anaesthetists.

By the turn of the millennium, however, the situation had

changed. Anaesthetists started providing care to patients not just in the operating theatre but also in other sectors of the hospital. They became involved in the pre-assessment before surgery, during the surgical operation as well as during post-operative care. Their role expanded to high dependency and intensive care, obstetric analgesia and anaesthesia, acute clinical episodes in emergency rooms, major accident management and resuscitation and for acute and chronic pain management. Within a few decades the anaesthetist transformed into an indispensible entity involved with the entire care pathway, from the beginning to the end. Anaesthesia of today is the science of understanding and correction of deranged body physiology in illness or injury – surgical or otherwise. The advances in anaesthesia were helped by the concomitant technological explosion during the last few decades, which helped in the advancement of sophisticated monitoring systems. These changes contributed to the overall development of safer surgical practice.

One of the memorable events of my career was to listen in person to the star surgeon of my lifetime – the famous, fluent and flamboyant Dr Christiaan Barnard – the man who made history and became the darling of the world overnight, which he acknowledged himself in the famous quote, "On Saturday, I was a surgeon in South Africa, very little known. On Monday, I was world renowned."

His arrival in India during the late seventies led to a frenzy of excitement throughout the country, despite the fact that the event that transformed him into a celebrity had happened more than a decade before. I was working as a urological resident at All India Institute of Medical Sciences, New Delhi, at that time and was one of the lucky ones to be allowed into the auditorium, whilst the streets outside were filled with crowds of people, press and police.

Here was a white man, born and raised in apartheid-ridden South Africa, addressing a predominantly non-white audience, talking about equality and diversity of the human race and emphasising repeatedly that black and white hearts have identical electrophysiology. Smooth, silky and smart, Barnard skilfully narrated the incredible story about the first heart transplant operation that he had performed on Louis Washkansky, a fifty-four year old grocer on 3 December 1967. The donor-heart came from a young woman named Denise Darvall, who had been rendered brain dead in an accident a day earlier while crossing a street in Cape Town. The patient survived only for a few days, but Dr Barnard's second patient lived for nineteen months.

The audience remained spellbound throughout as they heard the charismatic, well-attired and handsome Barnard – who could easily have replaced Sean Connery or Roger Moore as James Bond – deliver his speech with mesmerising precision, in delightful South African-English accent. In return, he received bouts of deafening applause from a packed house after every few sentences. It was patently obvious that the guy loved attention and enjoyed every moment of it.

The heart was the biggest prize for transplant surgeons and the event generated huge media interest. Following Barnard's bold leap, over a hundred heart transplants were performed in 1968-69, but almost all patients died within sixty days. However, the story of organ transplantation – one of the fascinating chapters of surgical advancement during the twentieth century, carried on. It must be said that surgeons received an unfairly larger share of glory and glamour; those who worked behind the scenes and changed the profile of transplantation from research to life-saving treatment deserved equal or perhaps more credit. Bruce Reitz who performed the first successful heart-lung transplant at Stanford in 1981 quite rightly credited the patient's recovery to the immunosuppressive drug cyclosporine-A and not to himself.

During my student days I had the opportunity of borrowing from a friend an old and partially torn copy of the fiction entitled *Brave New World*, by the British writer Aldous Huxley, published during the nineteen-thirties. The book starts off with a tour of a factory that produces human babies through methods of mass production. Natural birth did not exist; test tube reproduction had been perfected with the ability to divide the fertilised eggs to create up to ninety-six identical eggs from the original and mass produce identical workers with varied intelligence. As I started reading it, I found the fiction so unreal that after reading about half of the book I returned it to the owner without finishing the rest. At that time I thought that the book was a product of the author's disorderly imagination. How very foolish and wrong I was? Only a few years down the line, the world welcomed the first test tube baby – Louise Joy Brown – who was born in Oldham, UK on 25 July 1978. The media called her the super-babe.

The concept of the test tube baby – that involved the process of fertilisation of a human sperm and a human egg outside the human body – was again a triumphant endpoint to painstaking scientific research. The success story was no utopian fiction or miracle but a reality – an example of application of basic science to mysteries of nature. The story carries on: earlier this year the British Parliament voted for the creation of babies with DNA from two women and one man.

The boundless curiosity to look inside human cavities was instrumental in accelerating the development of modern surgical practice. At the beginning of my apprenticeship in India I had to learn the technique of looking inside a urinary bladder and inserting a plastic tube into the ureter (tubular conduit connecting the kidney to bladder), by using a solid metal cylindrical instrument that had a light bulb at the distal end for illuminating the bladder cavity. The trouble was that the bulb would not last long, and even if it did, with urine, water and sometimes blood around, the vision was so poor that my repeated attempts ended in failure. My frustration, which increased with each failed attempt, was augmented by the taunts of impatient anaesthetists and the ticking off from the theatre's chief nurse, who held me responsible for exhausting his stock of light bulbs. How could the boss do it so effortlessly and I couldn't? This was the vexing question that kept me awake for many nights, until one day I managed to negotiate the catheter successfully. Not only did all those present in theatre greet me with a loud cheer, but I also had to celebrate the achievement by hosting a departmental get-together.

However, we all were aware that there was light at the end of the tunnel and the future was much brighter because new instruments had been purchased by our hospital, which had already been shipped from Germany. The new system incorporated the Reading-based British physicist Harold Hopkins' inventions of coherent fibre-optics and rod-lens system, whereby light was transmitted through glass fibres and a series of lenses from an outside light source.

A few weeks after my hard-earned success with ureteral catheterization, the new set of instruments arrived, but to start with it was for use by the boss only – kids had to be content with window-shopping and we continued to toil with the older bulb model. When the restriction was eventually relaxed, one could suddenly see things. The surgeon's world had been illuminated – candlelight had been replaced by sunlight.

Hopkins' *Wave Theory of Aberrations* also provided the basis to modern optical design and gave the mathematical analysis that enabled the use of computers to create the high quality lenses available today.

Hopkins contributed hugely to the practice of modern surgery. The citation read at the time he received the medal from the Royal Society in 1984 stated, "In recognition of his many contributions to the theory and design of optical instruments, especially of a wide variety of important new medical instruments which have made a major contribution to clinical diagnosis and surgery."

The surgical maestro who removed my kidney stone during the late 1960s said to me, "I wish there was a way to make a small hole to pluck out the stone, but I am afraid there isn't," and as I made my way back after the consultation with him, his words resonated in my mind. I continued pondering about how one could make a small hole to pluck out the stone from the kidney. Many years down the line I found myself assisting John Wickham, a pioneer in the procedure of percutaneous nephrolithotomy (keyhole removal of a kidney stone) at the Institute of Urology, London for a similar sized stone as mine. On this occasion the patient went home next day with a 1cm size scar. In contrast, my inpatient stay was ten days and I was left with a 15cm-long scar.

Writing in the *BMJ* in 1987, Wickham coined the phrase 'minimally invasive surgery' and predicted that in the future open surgery would be limited to, "trauma and reconstruction," and that the next generation of surgeons would have to be trained as "microendoscopists and bioengineers rather than as butchers and carpenters".

The move from big cuts to keyholes was largely the result of technological advancement but, despite the availability of tools, the majority of surgical community was initially slow to embrace the idea. Gynaecologists and to a large extent urologists seized the opportunity at the dawn of the optical revolution. At the turn of the millennium when it finally took off, there was an explosion and within a few years minimally invasive surgery became widely available. The reign of the big surgeon making the big cut, who had ruled the surgical empire for more than a hundred years, came to an end as the keyhole surgeon took over. An Indian surgical colleague describes the transition in the following anecdote.

LEARNING THE HARD WAY (FROM CG, INDIA, 2005)

I had been working as a house officer on the general surgical firm for about a month at the teaching hospital. The registrar told me to excise a sebaceous cyst from a young lady's back. The patient had already been put to sleep, but the registrar had to go and attend an emergency on the ward.

I started the procedure without realising that the chief was standing behind me, and as I made a short but feeble cut on the top of the swelling, I heard him say, "Grow up into a man, make a longer and deeper cut! If you want to be a surgeon, remember that good surgeons are not scared to make big incisions."

Nervously, I extended and deepened the incision, following which he left the theatre and I carried on with the procedure.

About twenty years later, during a surgeon's conference in India, I was one of the trainers on a teaching course on laparoscopic cholecystectomy (keyhole removal of gall bladder). After the lectures, the next part of the course was hands-on training at various stations. A colleague and I moved from one station to another to teach the trainees and answer their questions.

At one of the stations an older-looking trainee, in his late fifties, asked me, "Do you recognise me?"

"No, I am sorry I don't but I must say your face looks familiar," I replied.

"You do not recognise me but you were my house surgeon," he said proudly and nervously while glancing at other people standing round the station.

In a flash I remembered him, his rigid surgical ways, his disciplined attitude to life and work, and his words: "… good surgeons are not scared to make big incisions." The man looked shorter and much older, and before I could utter anything he said, "I know what you are going to say, but you see times have changed. There is still some life left in me, so I must learn new techniques, even though it is hard to do that."

I am not sure if he remembered any of the words that he had articulated twenty years before. But the chance meeting made me think that the man who could whip out a gall bladder neatly by an open operation in thirty minutes and from whom I had learnt so many things had been honest to admit and accept the change in the surgical landscape.

I said, "Sir, I have pleasant memories of the time that I spent with you. You contributed hugely to whatever I am today. You are my guru, thank you so much."

In line with the improvements in technology and technical skills of surgeons, the list of laparoscopic procedures grew at an unprecedented pace in a short space of time. The loss of haptic (force and tactile) feedback and restricted degrees of instrument movement in laparoscopic surgery were accepted as drawbacks. The physiologic tremor in the surgeon's hand readily transmitted through the length of rigid instruments was an added problem. These limitations made delicate dissections and anastomoses tricky, but not impossible. The desire to overcome these and to expand the benefits of minimally invasive surgery, coupled with the development of concepts of telesurgery, were the motivating factors in the rapid development of robotic surgery.

Robotic surgery is the cocktail of the latest advances in robotics – computing, and medical imaging – that essentially puts a computer between the surgeon and the surgical tools operating on the patient. The instruments are mounted on the robotic arms introduced into the patient's body through keyholes. The surgeon's hand movements are scaled and filtered to eliminate hand tremor, then translated into micro-movements of the proprietary instruments. The camera used in the system provides a true stereoscopic picture that is transmitted to a surgeon's console. Surgeons don't move endoscopic instruments directly with their hands. Instead, they sit at a console several feet from the operating table and use joysticks similar to those used in video games. They perform surgical tasks by guiding the movement of the robotic arms in a process known as tele-manipulation.

Robots have superhuman capabilities; they do not tire. Moreover, robotic arms have a wide range of movement and remain steady at all times that makes it easier for surgeons to manipulate tissues and work from difficult angles, and operate in parts of the body where human hands can't reach. Robotic surgical systems also improve depth perception and provide surgeons with haptic feedback and three-dimensional vision, compared with the two-dimensional view they normally get with the endoscopic procedures. The surgical field can be magnified so that millimetre-sized vessels appear as big as pencils. Compared with the long instruments used in endoscopy, robotic surgical systems use smaller instruments that provide an increased range of motion. What humans can't do, computerised systems can!

Robotic telesurgery has been flaunted as a geographic long jump – a solution to surgical problems in the developing world, whereby a single central hospital can operate several remote machines at distant locations. It has strong military application too; it can provide mobile care to the injured, and keep trained clinical staff safe from the battle zone. An obstacle in telesurgery is the delay of movement – the latency between the surgeon moving his hands, to the robotic arms responding to those movements. As scientists, technicians and entrepreneurs work through these difficulties and improve the robotic systems with supersensitive haptic technology and find ways to reduce the costs involved, in time expert surgical treatment by robotic surgery will become available at remote places in the world where it never reached before.

Notwithstanding the fact that I was nurtured during the glory days of open surgery, I was convinced quite early that the direction of the surgical journey would shift from an open cut to a keyhole. However, I could never imagine that robotic surgery would explode on the scene so rapidly.

Multifaceted advances in science and technology – physics, genetics, stem cell research, engineering, information technology, Internet etc. – have had a phenomenal impact on every aspect of human life and behaviour. Surgeons and surgical practice are no exceptions. With the discovery of the genetic code and its function on protein synthesis, for which the researchers were awarded the

Nobel Prize, prevention and cure of disease by molecular surgical tools rather than by surgical operations became possible and will in time become a routine. As science solves the riddle of ageing, the whole profile of surgical practice is bound to transform in the years to come. Stem cell development and innovations in physics and technology will combine to produce bodily parts – organs, joints and limbs – possibly brains or even bionic entities.

Earlier this year the Star Robot, that doesn't need to be controlled by surgeon's hands, was used successfully to stich together a pig's bowel and the performance matched to that of trained doctors. As the concept of a robot undertaking a surgical procedure independently on a human being becomes a reality, in the brave new world the surgeon could become an antiquated entity. At best the human surgeon may find a role like the conductor of an orchestra – working on a keyboard in a large office, directing a pack of androids – the surgical workers of the future.

But does it matter whether the surgeon is a man or a machine? Imagine a situation where you are seated in a chair, or lying wide-awake on the operating table within the premises of a High Street care provider, and the automaton starts working on the anaesthetised part of your body. And if you fancy some more work on another part of your body, or wish to have a haircut, manicure, pedicure or facial (or all of these) on the same day, all you may have to do is to tap a couple of keys on the keyboard and change the program, so that the same robotic hands perform different tasks.

But what if one is blown up into the clouds in a state of slumber by an anaesthetic cocktail and the human directing the action hits the wrong key; or what if during the surgical voyage the automaton is challenged by something it has never confronted before? When the academics busily working on 'artificial intelligence', are able to create computers and computer software capable of intelligent and independent thinking and behaviour, just like the human, the humanoid would be able to steer the helm and follow the right course. And there may not be even the need for a human to push the buttons or tap the keys. My imagination may be running wild, but it's hard to believe how far I have travelled from the good old times of the *naevid* (barber-surgeon) in such a short time.

ACKNOWLEDGEMENTS

I would like to thank every clinician who took the time to respond to my request for surgical anecdotes. I received a large number of these but for various reasons couldn't incorporate all in this book and I apologise to colleagues whose material could not be included.

I am thankful to everyone who assisted in the editing and proofreading. The first person to read the initial draft of the manuscript a couple of years ago was my friend Mr Peter Cook (ex-medical correspondent of the Kent Messenger Group of Newspapers). His suggestions were enormously valuable in shaping the final version.

I am grateful to my surgical colleague and the President of my association (British Association of Urological Surgeons), Mr Mark Speakman for reading the manuscript and writing a foreword.

My thanks are also due to Mr Ronald Hoile consultant surgeon for allowing me to use his original painting for the front cover of the book.

Spending so much time on my laptop in my little study, I am lucky to have a trusted and dear soul mate – my wife Razia, who was there with words of encouragement, cups of tea and ideas. Days spent on writing this book actually belonged to her.

My advisors – my sons Arjmand and Iqbal and their spouses Sehla & Ayesha, who have read the book without reading it, were always there to talk things over.

Thanks also go to Mr Aadil Khan – the only budding surgeon in our large family of many doctors, for the surgical chats that we both enjoy during our family get-togethers.

Finally, I am obliged to everyone at Book Guild & Company, for being so understanding and patient.